The Functions of Sleep

The Functions of Sleep

ERNEST L. HARTMANN, M.D.

New Haven and London, Yale University Press, 1973

Library of Congress catalog card number: 73-79983
International standard book number: 0-300-01700-6 (cloth);
0-300-01701-4 (paper)

Designed by Sally Sullivan
and set in Times Roman (CRT) type.
Printed in the United States of America by
The Colonial Press Inc., Clinton, Massachusetts

Published in Great Britain, Europe, and Africa by
Yale University Press, Ltd., London.
Distributed in Latin America by Kaiman & Polon,
Inc., New York City; in Australasia and Southeast
Asia by John Wiley & Sons Australasia Pty. Ltd.,
Sydney; in India by UBS Publishers' Distributors Pvt.,
Ltd., Delhi; in Japan by John Weatherhill, Inc., Tokyo.

43971

For
Jonathan and Katie

Contents

Acknowledgments

I am happy to acknowledge my major debts to both organizations and individuals. I am sincerely grateful to the Association for the Psychophysiological Study of Sleep for the guidance and the sense of togetherness it has brought to the field of sleep research; to the National Institute of Mental Health for the money it has provided, usually very equitably in my opinion, to researchers including myself in this field; and to the Countway Library, Boston, and the Brain Information Service, Los Angeles, for rapid access to essential information.

Specifically, I should like to thank Drs. Jonathan Cole, Jack Ewalt, Charles Fisher, Ramon Greenberg, Milton Greenblatt, Dora Hartmann, Larry Hartmann, David Hawkins, J. Allan Hobson, Anton Kris, William Meissner, Chester Pearlman, Myron Sharaf, James Skinner, Leonard Solomon, and George Vaillant for reading and commenting on this manuscript or earlier papers on which it is based.

I am grateful to Drs. Frederick Baekeland, Ching-piao Chien, Richard Chung, Paul Draskoczy, Mechte Papoucek, Sid Perzow, Charles Popper, Joseph Schildkraut, Warren Stern, and Robert Watson for their collaboration on certain of the studies on which this book is based. I wish to thank Tom Amatruda, Sarah Auchincloss, Jacob Bernstein, Valarie Brewer, Denny Bridwell, James Cravens, Carol Galginaitis, Susan Koski, Sam List, Herbie Marsden, Ellen Moran, Ann Owens, Karen-Lee Rosenthal, Gail Stanford, Susan Wise, and George Zwilling for their assistance, collaboration, and support (i.e. honest-to-goodness work) in our sleep laboratory studies. I am aware particularly that I could not have managed without James Cravens and George Zwilling, though I sometimes think they might have managed quite well without me.

Finally, I am indebted to my dedicated secretary, Pat Sullivan, who, with the help of a few illegible scribbles and inaudible recordings, wrote this book.

I. INTRODUCTION AND PREVIOUS THEORIES

1 Introduction

This book will attempt two tasks and will inevitably fall short of perfection in each. First, after considering previous theories of the function of sleep and reviewing recent sleep research, I shall present my own theory arrived at through a number of very different lines of evidence. Second, I hope this effort may serve as a prototype for other studies of mind-body relationships. Focusing on a specific goal—explaining the functional role of sleep—I shall attempt to show that evidence derived from chemistry and pharmacology, from neurophysiology, from simple observational studies of behavior, and from psychoanalysis can all, with perhaps a touch of speculative nudging, converge on the same general formulation. Further, I shall try to demonstrate that this convergence explains a great deal of already existing information in simple terms and, in addition, suggests whole areas for future exploration, since it implies a theory of the chemical and neural mechanisms responsible for important aspects of mental functioning.

In sleep research, as in other areas of scientific inquiry, *why* is often the first question asked and the last question answered, or left unanswered. To the layman, Why do we sleep? is a natural question, and he even has an answer, though in very vague terms: sleep restores. The scientist usually retreats from the question, considering it either unscientific or too large to tackle. Some scientists feel that their job is to study only mechanisms, or the *how,* and not functions, the *why.* Others, following Sherrington (1906), have a larger view of science: "Physiology pursues analysis of the reactions of the body considered as physical and chemical events; but, further, it aims at giving a reasoned account of the acts of an organism in respect of their purpose and use to the organism *qua* organism."

An inquiry into function or purpose has frequently been neglected or regarded with suspicion because of its historical connection with religion or with the search for a "higher purpose." Scientists have been rightly concerned when such a quest for purpose has substituted for a scientific inquiry into mechanism. However, the danger of this substitution is obviously not great at present, and the question of higher purpose really arises only when one is dealing with the highest level of organization—What is the function of man? What is the function of the universe?

I see the question of mechanism versus function, in a biological system at least, as a question of level of organization. When we ask *how,* we are studying mechanisms and we look at subunits (to discover how the kidney works one looks at the glomeruli and tubules). When we ask *why,* we are studying function and we look at larger systems (to study the function of the kidney one examines changes in blood chemistry and their effects on all systems of the body). Thus, for an intermediate system, the question of function is simply the question of a functional role in a larger system. For instance, it is clear that the function (or at least a function) of the kidney is to maintain a balance in blood chemistry by removing certain chemicals and that this plays a role in the survival of the larger entity, the body. Furthermore, awareness of this function helps rather than hinders more detailed research. For instance, laboratory and clinical studies of kidney abnormalities or dysfunction can be more precise, and one can now predict and study changes produced in other body systems by poor renal function. Renal physiology has advanced far beyond the stage of studying gross effects of total "kidney deprivation."

In my opinion there is no doubt that the function of sleep represents an important research question. The doubt is only whether enough information is available to attack the question properly and, of course, whether the proposals advanced here provide at least partial answers. This the reader now, tentatively, and further experiments later, more definitively, will have to decide.

There are some possible reasons for *not* studying the functions of sleep. First, there is the possibility that searching for functions of sleep may be a futile and even misleading enterprise. One interesting position is taken by Nathaniel Kleitman and a number of other sleep researchers. Kleitman's excellent and comprehensive review of sleep (1963) has 4,000 references and numerous chapters and subheadings covering what would seem to be all aspects of sleep, but the function or functions of sleep are never mentioned in the text or in the index. Kleitman does not discuss the question of function directly, nor does he discuss reasons for leaving it out. However, his publications and contributions to discussions of sleep make it clear that in his view sleep is a natural background state of the organism and of the brain, and it is meaningless to speak of its function. What needs to be studied, in Kleitman's view, are the departures from this state—the mechanisms and functions of wakefulness.

Even though I do not object to the study of wakefulness (in fact most of biology, insofar as it has any concern for behavior, has consisted of studies of wakefulness), I cannot accept this point of view. Actually there is much recent evidence, to be reviewed later (chapter 3), that sleep is by no means an inactive state for the nervous system, but this is not the essential point. To my mind it makes little sense to consider sleep either more or less natural than wakefulness; however, taking the functional point of view, it is obvious that the eventual functions to be served—survival of the individual and of the species—involve tasks which are carried out during wakefulness: eating, mating, rearing one's young, and all the many complex maneuvers preparatory to these. Proper waking functioning directed toward these goals is obviously essential for the organism; and it would be reasonable to suppose that if sleep has a function, it might play a role in the optimal functioning of the state of wakefulness. The contrary argument—that waking is necessary to insure optimal sleep— obviously cannot be made. Therefore, without assigning any priority or greater naturalness to either state, I believe it is entirely justifiable to search for functions of sleep and to expect that these functions when discovered will involve maintenance of the waking state optimal, directly or indirectly, for preservation of the individual and the species.

There is another group of researchers who insist that it is futile to look for specific functions for such a solid, stable, and difficult-to-alter part of the mammalian organism as sleep. Indeed, Webb's group has presented considerable evidence of the solidity of sleep-waking cycles and of the great difficulty of producing long-term changes in the sleep patterns of animals under a variety of apparently powerful experimental conditions (Webb and Friedman 1971; Webb 1961, 1969). The argument is that if various environmental "demands" produce little change in sleep time, sleep cannot be performing much of a function in answering these demands, and thus sleep once more is relegated to a sort of background which merely exists as part of an overall sleep-wake cycle, a cycle which itself is then presumed to have an adaptive role.

I have two objections to this point of view, although I would agree that a possible functional role for the overall sleep-wake cycle should be kept in mind in addition to a functional role of sleep. First, the fact that it is difficult to alter the amount of sleep in a stable fashion by experimental manipulations (difficult but not impossible, as will be discussed further on) does not indicate that sleep cannot have a function, even a specific restorative function with regard to certain daytime activities. It may simply be that the normal amount of sleep is sufficient in most individuals to handle a considerable range of waking activity that might require restoration. There may, in other words, be a large "reserve" which makes it difficult to produce overall changes. And, furthermore, gross change in the amount of sleep may not be the essential variable. The various organs of the body fulfill their functions over a wide range of demands without gross changes in size or configuration, but one often finds some change when one examines the relevant substructures or physiological variables, such as arterial and venous pH or levels of blood metabolites, rather than looking at the size of the lungs or kidneys. Thus, in situations where no gross change in amount of sleep is found, it is still worth looking at details of the substructure of sleep and various neural or behavioral variables before and after sleep. In fact there is some evidence, to be reviewed, that certain aspects of the structure of sleep can be changed under different waking conditions, which may represent different demands for restoration by sleep.

If one does accept the legitimacy of looking for functions of sleep, there is a further question as to whether one should expect one function for such a complex entity as sleep, or a whole series of functions, or perhaps two separate series of functions for the two sleep states, *synchronized* (S) and *desynchronized* (D) sleep (see chapter 3).[1] I have previously taken the position that since sleep or in fact S- and D-sleep are each major states in many ways on a par with wakefulness, one might expect such a complex array of functions on chemical, physiological, and psychological levels that it would be almost futile to speak of *the* function of sleep (1967). Indeed I have titled the present effort "the function*s* of sleep" with this point in mind. However, after many experiments and reformulations, I have recently come to the conclusion that the problem is not hopeless after all, that it is possible to arrive at one broad function for S-sleep and one for D-sleep, and that the two functions are closely linked, as indeed the two states are linked in sleep. Although the functions of sleep can be looked at and examined differently from chemical,

1. Almost all researchers now recognize the presence of two qualitatively different states of mammalian sleep: One is associated with a relative slowing of the EEG, general quiescence of the autonomic nervous system, no rapid eye movements, and thoughtlike mental activity; this is called S (synchronized) sleep, NREM (non-rapid-eye-movement) sleep, or orthodox sleep. The other is associated with a desynchronized EEG, activation of the autonomic nervous system and portions of the central nervous system, rapid eye movements, and typical dream reports; this is called D (desynchronized or dreaming) sleep, REM sleep, or paradoxical sleep.

physiological, or psychological perspectives, and this work will range widely, though I hope not wildly, among these disciplines, I shall attempt to show that evidence from all these directions can lead to a coherent view of the overall function of sleep.

2 Theories of the Functions of Sleep

Space will not permit detailed discussion of the older theories of the function of sleep, but the reader may note that some of these theories formulated, in terms appropriate to their times, ideas similar to those of more recent theories including the one to be developed here. Aside from this conclusion that there is nothing truly new under the sun, consideration of the older views of function will not lead us far, since they are hardly ever formulated in terms amenable to meaningful experimentation by present methods. This unfortunate fate of many theories should, I suppose, strike at least caution if not terror into the hearts of those of us who are still trying.

I shall then consider more recent theories of function, which often discuss separately the functions of two states of sleep or restrict themselves to the function of one state. The reader who is not familiar with some of the terms and concepts used will find it easier to skip this section and to return to it after reading chapter 3, which briefly summarizes recent sleep research.

Some early theories saw sleep as a means of preventing or combating fatigue. Claparède (1908) suggests that sleep functions to prevent fatigue, *épuisement,* and that sleep has a specific restorative function in "balancing wakefulness . . . because in sleep mental tension is replaced by a vegetative tension." He does not specify exactly what requires balancing. Coriat (1912) also proposes that sleep is a reactionary defense of the organism against fatigue. (He gives some physical aspects of it which are difficult to follow.)

Hess (1929, 1931*a*, 1931*b*) suggests that sleep is a vegetative homeostatic system, in which the trophotropic mechanisms of the nervous system take over and provide restitution (no details are supplied) after the predominance of the ergotropic mechanisms during waking. "At the height of maximal activity the vegetative functions cannot keep pace with the demands of the moment and a negative balance ensues in the required equilibrium between somatic and autonomic functions. With the onset of fatigue a re-establishment of that equilibrium is introduced" (1965). He does not clearly differentiate between what needs to be restored by sleep and what can be restored by inactive wakefulness.

The great neurologist Hughlings Jackson made no particular study of sleep but nonetheless proposes an interesting function (1932). He relates sleep to memory and suggests that sleep functions both to sweep away unnecessary memories and connections from the day and perhaps to consolidate or maintain more necessary ones. This anticipates a number of more recent hypotheses, as will be seen, and there is some evidence from studies of sleep deprivation and of sleep effects on memory and learning that can be seen as supporting Jackson's general formulation.

One view of sleep which has had numerous proponents and opponents is that an energy deficit, or oxygen debt, builds up during waking and is compensated for during sleep (Wohlisch 1956; and reviewed in Koella 1967). However, careful studies of cerebral oxygen consumption have found no differences in oxygen consumption between sleeping and waking states.[1]

Pavlov (1952; Cuny 1962) states that sleep is the irradiation of inhibition throughout the cortex. Portions of the cortex which remain excited during sleep account for dreaming. He notes that sleep can be brought on by either a decrease in stimulation or an excess of stimulation, and in terms of function he suggests that the balance of the excitation-inhibition continuum is protected by sleep. These views lend themselves to experimental examination to a certain extent. At least the idea of cortical inhibition can be examined, and indeed cortical neurons do tend to fire less during sleep, or at least during S-sleep, than during waking. However, the statement that sleep functions to protect the excitation-inhibition continuum is harder to pin down and test. Insofar as

1. Mangold, Sokoloff, Conner, Kleinerman, Therman, and Kety 1955.

Pavlov's meaning is that incoming stimuli are handled differently during sleep, he is probably right, and this may be a kind of "protection" for the brain. Also, if by "excitation-inhibition continuum" he means something like general homeostasis for the brain, his formulation may well find support.

Sigmund Freud (1953), who had much to say about possible functions of dreaming, gives only rough hints of his ideas on the functions of sleep. He suggests, using the topographic model of the psyche (conscious, preconscious, and unconscious), that it is primarily the preconscious which requires sleep. Furthermore, since what he calls intrapsychic censorship is relaxed during sleep, allowing the emergence of unconscious repressed material in the dream, he hints that one function of sleep might be to allow such emergence with consequent drive discharge. Freud goes no further, and in fact specifically states that the function of sleep will probably turn out to be a biological rather than a psychological problem.

After Freud, some psychoanalysts, interested primarily in dreams, invoked Freud's formulation of a "wish to sleep." This is especially prominent in Lewin (1950), for whom the "dream screen," the background matrix which he sees behind all dreams, represents this wish to sleep. Proponents of these views see sleep as a blissful return to the breast or to the womb, serving a sort of symbolic function in the organization of the psyche, but they do not, I believe, claim this as the entire explanation of the functional role of sleep. It can also be inferred that sleep functions as an important regression in the service of the ego. Aside from this, classical psychoanalysts have had relatively little to say about the functions of sleep, although I would suggest that careful psychoanalytic explorations of the functioning of the waking mind might provide a useful approach to exactly what mechanisms or processes require the restoration that might be provided by sleep; this is an approach which I shall take up later.

Many of these theories are imaginative and make a certain

amount of sense, but I am not certain that they take us much beyond the well-known views of an early seventeenth-century sleep investigator, who describes "sleep, chief nourisher at life's feast" and "sleep, which knits up the raveled sleave of care" (Shakespeare 1623). In fact, we will see that these two descriptions may turn out to be excellent guesses.

In recent years, since the discovery of two separate states of sleep, S and D—which will be discussed at length in the next chapter—there has been a large amount of empirical research with but a few attempts at delineating function. The few attempts available have tended to refer specifically to one or the other sleep state. The D-state, or rapid-eye-movement sleep, because of its association with dreaming, has especially interested a number of workers.

Several theories suggest, along with Pavlov and others, that one part of sleep, most probably S-sleep, has a difficult-to-specify function of pure rest or inactivity for cortical neurons; they then propose that the other phase of sleep, D-sleep, functions to interrupt this state of quiescence. Thus Ephron and Carrington (1966) have suggested that S-sleep is a kind of sensory deprivation or cortical deafferentation which may be necessary (for unspecified reasons), but that long periods of such deprivation may be dangerous. They then suggest that D-sleep is a homeostatic mechanism whose role is to "reaffer-ent" the cortex—bring the level of cortical excitation back to some necessary level. Similarly, Weiss (1966) has suggested that D-sleep functions to reorganize central nervous system (CNS) firing patterns which have become somehow disorganized during S-sleep, and Hawkins (1966) has suggested that D-sleep serves "to regularly reestablish patterned operation."

Related to this is Snyder's hypothesis of the "arousal function" of D-sleep (1966). His view, based to a great extent on phylogenetic considerations and the large amounts of sleep found in some primitive mammals, is that sleep as a whole functions to conserve energy (i.e. a sleeping animal uses up less energy than a waking animal) and also functions, in certain species at least, to keep the animal out of harm's way for a good portion of the 24 hours. With this as an overall function for sleep, Snyder then suggests that an animal sleeping for too many hours may be in danger from predators, and so a periodic arousal mechanism is useful, and this is the role played by the recurrent D-periods, which indeed do have certain characteristics of cortical arousal. This theory is consistent with the fact that in many species a brief arousal tends to follow each D-period. However, one cannot help thinking that this theory would better explain a state of affairs in which S-sleep was simply interrupted by brief periodic arousals rather than involving the intricacies of the D-state; and what is hardest to reconcile with the theory is that during D-sleep, despite the "aroused-looking" recordings from its cortex, the animal actually has a higher arousal threshold to external stimulation than during S-sleep (Benoit and Bloch 1960; Dillon and Webb 1965).[2]

Hawkins (1966) has proposed a formulation similar to Snyder's hypothesis but along psychoanalytic lines, that there is a need for the ego to be periodically recathected and that this occurs during dreaming periods.

Also related to the afferentation or cortical excitation view of D-sleep is a theory of the functions of desynchronized sleep derived from ontogenetic data by Roffwarg, Muzio, and Dement (1966). These authors are struck especially by the large amounts and high percentages of D-time found in young or newborn animals and the likelihood that even higher percentages are found in utero. Citing evidence that a certain amount of stimulation is necessary for the proper development of the mammalian cortex, they suggest that the newborn mammal sleeps a great deal and has need of more

2. There are a number of studies in this area, and though all agree that arousal thresholds are generally higher in D-sleep than in S-sleep, some have found exceptions, e.g. lower or equally low thresholds in D-sleep when an auditory stimulus was "familiar" or "significant" to the animal or human subject. But surely if D-sleep has an arousal function, it would be especially important that the animal be easily aroused by unfamiliar or unknown sounds.

stimulation to the cortex than can be provided by sensory stimulation from the outside during waking; hence the D-periods, which provide a sort of endogenous, quasi-sensory neural bombardment of the cortex. The fetus, of course, with almost no "external" stimulation, would have even greater need of such endogenous stimulation.

Then there are a number of related theories proposing that sleep, especially D-sleep, has a role in dealing with memory and learning. The simplest of these, based on a superficial view of dream content and a computer analogy, suggests that D-sleep functions merely to clear the tapes of irrelevant information gathered during the daytime so that new information may be absorbed the next day (Newman and Evans 1965). This role corresponds to one-half of the functions that Hughlings Jackson proposed—sweeping away useless memories and consolidating useful ones. The notion that sleep or D-sleep has a role in consolidating useful memories has also had a number of proponents. Breger (1967) has suggested that D-sleep and dreaming are especially necessary for a kind of learning or memory consolidation which he calls "perceptual learning."

Moruzzi (1966) suggests that sleep permits recovery of "plastic synapses" in the brain and plays a role in the formation of engrams. Gaarder (1966) has similarly proposed that memories may be processed and coded during D-sleep. Hennevin and Leconte (1971), after an extensive review, also suggest an information-handling and memory-consolidation function for D.

Dewan (1969, 1970) proposes what he calls the "programming" hypothesis—that during sleep, and especially during dreaming sleep, there is a reprogramming going on. Although some programming can occur during waking, certain broad or emotion-containing programs or perhaps higher-level "metaprograms" need to be elaborated during sleep.

Greenberg and Pearlman (1972) hold somewhat similar views—that D-sleep is involved in reprogramming the brain, especially in the integration of new experiences with existing personality. Greenberg and Leiderman (1966) believe that D-sleep may involve rewinding recent memories onto long-term storage tapes. These workers suggest that the memories handled during dreaming are those which are especially emotional and that a function of D-sleep is to repress, to keep from waking consciousness, material that is arousing or threatening.[3] Pearlman speaks of these functions as a process of "emotional adaptation" (1970).

It is intriguing that so many investigators have come up with similar theories in recent years. And in fact the theory to be developed later in this work involves aspects of memory and learning functions as well. That sleep should have some such function is certainly believable, although evidence is as yet not entirely convincing. Evidence relating to these functions will be mentioned in later chapters.

Another theory related to learning is that of Feinberg and Evarts (1969a), which is based almost entirely on age curves—distribution of sleep and of the D-state with age—and the changes produced when mental functioning is very poor. They hold that sleep, especially D-sleep, bears a general relationship to intellectual ability, since D-sleep is lower when intellectual function or ability is low (see chapter 7).

There are several theories on a biological level which do not fit even roughly into either the deafferentation and reafferentation model or the learning and memory models. Berger (1969), for example, proposes that D-sleep has a function in restoring the neuronal and neuromuscular apparatus necessary for binocular vision. To support his hypothesis, he cites indirect correlations between amount of decussation of the optic tracts, related to binocular vision, with amount of D-time across species, and he has recently provided some experimental evidence as well; but conflicting evidence also exists (Herman, Tauber, Rosenman, and Roffwarg 1971).

Dement and several others have suggested, on the basis of

3. Greenberg, Pearlman, Fingar, Kantrowitz, and Kawliche 1970.

a buildup and discharge model of desynchronized sleep, that D-sleep may function periodically to clear the central nervous system of some endogenous substance or toxin that builds up during waking and during S-sleep (Dement 1964). This is possible, but it does not explain the complex nature of D-sleep which especially Dement and his collaborators have been so carefully elucidating.

An intriguing theory proposed by Freemon (1970) suggests that there are two arousal systems and that the continued need for vigilance, employing two separate systems, accounts for the presence of two separate sleep states. The evidence is mainly neuroanatomical—there are slow waves in one system when there are fast waves in the other. This appears to me to be an auxiliary theory which does not actually tackle function: whatever function sleep serves, which Freemon simply refers to as "renewal," the animal must be protected by at least a rudimentary vigilance system; he is simply suggesting two separate vigilance systems, one for S and one for D.

Fisher (1965a, 1965b) has accepted to a certain extent Freud's view that dreams, and thus presumably the D-state, have a function in discharging instinctual drives in the adult. He believes that in the child, where true instinctual drives may not be present in the same sense, the D-state functions to discharge "physiological" drives. This view is consistent with the buildup and discharge aspect of the sleep-dream cycle, which many authors have commented on and which may characterize the entire life of the newborn and very young child (Wolff 1966). It is also consistent with the fact that D-deprivation may produce hungry and hypersexual cats (Dement 1970), but otherwise it is a very difficult theory to support or refute experimentally.

Spitz, Emde, and Metcalf (1970) have proposed a function specifically for S-sleep, without bothering about D which appears to have fascinated most of their colleagues. Based entirely on a study showing that S-sleep was greatly increased after the stress of neonatal circumcision, they suggest that S may have a "conservation-withdrawal" function in the neonate, and this form of sleep may be a prototype for later psychic patterns of defense. Again conservation-withdrawal is attractive but not very specific.

Finally, French, Jones, and a number of others have suggested some specific functions of dreaming as a means of mastering current problems and conflicts and thus achieving better psychological adaptation for future waking life.[4] The implication is that sleep as a whole, or at least D-sleep, allows the process of dreaming, which in turn has the adaptational function mentioned.

I believe that many of these theories of function contain at least kernels of truth. Most do not seem to provide a view of function proportionate to what we know of the complexity or the beauty of the sleep cycles. Perhaps I am introducing aesthetic principles out of place, but while awaiting further evidence on the binocular vision hypothesis or the arousal hypothesis, I nonetheless feel that these are at best incomplete theories. Even if true, they do not account for the intricacies of sleep—the regular cycling, the almost invariant relations between the two states, the specific neurological events, and the dream. And, in general, these theories are derived from and tested on very delimited areas of research.

I shall now attempt to derive a theory of the functions of sleep by a process of convergence from a number of different starting points, to be taken up in chapters 3 through 12. First, hints as to function that can be derived from a review of the large body of recent research on the physiology and chemistry of sleep will be explored. Next we shall approach functions of sleep through the psychological and physiological effects of sleep deprivation, and of deprivation of the two important states of sleep: dreaming or desynchronized sleep (D) and synchronized sleep (S). Then we shall take up certain

4. French and Fromm 1964; Jones 1962; Garma 1966; Wolff 1952; Maeder 1916.

relevant experiments in nature: What are the psychological characteristics of "long sleepers" and "short sleepers," persons who appear to require much more or much less sleep than the average? And a similar question will be asked of "variable sleepers": What characterizes periods with different sleep needs in persons whose sleep need varies greatly at different times? Next we shall consider functions of sleep by looking at *sleep as a response* (what "stimuli" or independent variables can affect sleep or sleep requirement): How does sleep respond to age, to pathological conditions, and to various behavioral, physiological, and chemical interventions? Then we shall see whether a psychological examination of the state of tiredness can give us insights as to functions of sleep, and finally we shall try to derive hints as to sleep functions by an examination of the structure of the dream. After summarizing a theory of the functions of sleep derived from all these directions, I shall end by suggesting some implications of this work for the scientific study of the brain and mind.

II. APPROACHES TO THE
FUNCTIONS OF SLEEP

3 Recent Sleep Research

This chapter will attempt to summarize some salient features of recent sleep research. The review will obviously not be complete; a review written in 1966 included 650 references (Hartmann 1967), and there would have to be several thousand by this time; rather, I shall emphasize what to my mind are the most important and accepted findings of recent sleep research. These findings should be encompassed by or at least clearly compatible with any theory of sleep function. Some fascinating but tentative lines of inquiry may be omitted if they are not relevant to the question of function.[1]

Definition of Sleep

First, it will be useful to keep in mind that, despite the fact that we shall speak to a great extent of EEG and polygraphic studies, sleep is not an EEG tracing but a behavioral state. One might define sleep as a recurrent, easily reversible condition characterized by relative quiescence and by a greatly increased threshold for response to external stimulation. Over the years, we have repeatedly found this behavioral state to be associated with certain patterns on the electroencephalogram, and these have gradually become known as EEG sleep patterns. However, I have no doubt that if I found a person walking and talking rationally to me while I recorded "EEG sleep patterns" from his brain, I would question the adequacy of our EEG definitions rather than insist that despite appearances he was actually asleep. This is not solely of academic interest, since EEG patterns usually associated with sleep may indeed be found during waking

1. The reader who wishes more complete information or more extensive references may want to refer to several recent books summarizing sleep research (Koella 1967; Hartmann 1970a; Freemon 1972) or to the most comprehensive text available on sleep (Kleitman 1963).

under certain drug conditions, and likewise patterns usually associated with sleep can be found during anesthesia or coma.

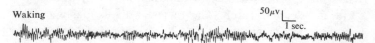

Figure 1. The EEG of sleep in a human adult. A single channel of recording—a monopolar recording from the left parietal area, referred to the ears as a neutral reference point—is shown for each stage.

The EEG of Sleep

As the subject falls asleep on a clinical EEG table, his brain waves go through certain characteristic changes, often classified arbitrarily into four stages (see figure 1). The waking EEG is characterized by alpha waves (8–12 cycles per second) and low-voltage activity of mixed frequency. As a subject falls asleep, his alpha rhythm often disappears and reappears a few times and then is gradually lost. Stage 1, which is considered the lightest stage of sleep, is characterized by low-voltage, desynchronized activity and sometimes by low-voltage, regular 4–6-cycles-per-second activity as well. After a few seconds or minutes this gives way to stage 2, a pattern characterized chiefly by frequent 13–15-cycles-per-second spindle-shaped tracings, known as sleep spindles, and by certain high-voltage spikes known as *K-complexes*. In a few more minutes delta waves, higher-voltage activity at 1–4 cycles per second, make their appearance (stage 3), and eventually these delta waves occupy the major part of the record (stage 4).[2] The changes occurring during the onset of sleep can be recorded from almost anywhere on the scalp, although waking alpha is most prominent in the occipital areas, while the sleep spindles are more prominent in the parietal areas.

Two States of Sleep

Since the work of Aserinsky and Kleitman (1953, 1955), it has gradually become recognized that a night of sleep does not consist, as was thought for some years, of a transition from waking to deep slow waves (stage 4) and then back to waking. Rather, sleep is cyclical, with four or five periods of "emergence" from stages 2, 3, and 4 to something like stage 1 (see figure 2), but often containing small amounts of slow (8–10 cycles/sec) alpha activity and occasionally slower "sawtooth" waves. These four or five periods during the night are not typical stage 1 such as is found at sleep onset; in fact they are so different from the remainder of sleep, in many

2. Although the progression from stage 1 to stage 4 of S-sleep is actually a continuous process, the classification roughly sketched here has become quite standard. Details of the scoring can be found in Rechtschaffen and Kales (1968).

ways which will be described below, that they are now almost universally seen as constituting a separate "state" of sleep. This view is reinforced by the fact that similar periods, differing markedly from the remainder of sleep, are found in almost all mammals and in birds, as will be discussed. We refer to these periods of desynchronized sleep as D- (for desynchronized or dreaming) sleep and the remainder of sleep as S- (synchronized) sleep. These same two states are elsewhere referred to as REM (rapid eye movement) sleep and NREM (non–rapid eye movement) sleep, as paradoxical sleep and orthodox sleep, or as active sleep and quiet sleep.

The two states of sleep differ even behaviorally. In the adult human simple observation reveals few differences, although the careful observer may notice rapid movements of the eyes during D-periods and no such movements during S. An observer watching a young child sleep will notice a great many eye movements as well as movements of the small facial muscles which occur during D-periods, whereas whole-body jerks or simply quiescence characterize S-sleep.[3]

When physiological measurements are taken, further differences can be noted. Pulse and respiration are relatively low and steady during S-sleep but are somewhat faster and more irregular, at least in man, during D (Snyder, Hobson, Morrison, and Goldfrank 1964). Similarly, blood pressure is low and regular during S and somewhat higher and more irregular during D.[4] Penile erections have been found to be associated with almost all D-periods in the human male with little clear relationship to the nature of dream content.[5] Some neurophysiological studies of the two states will be discussed later.

The muscular system also shows interesting differences. It

3. Aserinsky and Kleitman 1955; Prechtl 1970; Parmelee, Schulz, and Disbrow 1961.
4. Snyder, Hobson, Morrison, and Goldfrank 1964; Williams and Cartwright 1969.
5. Fisher, Gross, and Zuch 1965; Karacan, Goodenough, Shapiro, and Starker 1966.

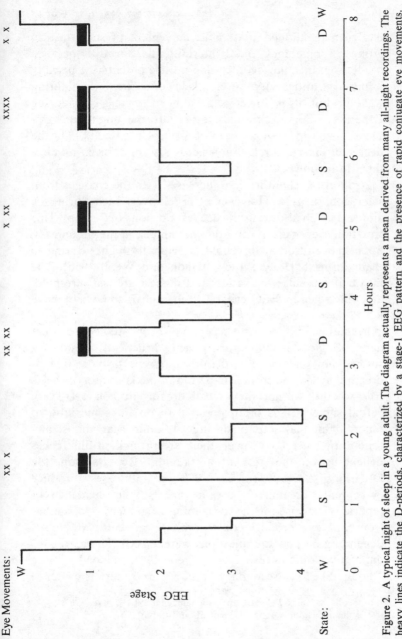

Figure 2. A typical night of sleep in a young adult. The diagram actually represents a mean derived from many all-night recordings. The heavy lines indicate the D-periods, characterized by a stage-1 EEG pattern and the presence of rapid conjugate eye movements. Reprinted from Hartmann (1967). W = waking; S = synchronized sleep; D = desynchronized or dreaming sleep.

has been mentioned that rapid movement of small-muscle groups is sometimes found intermittently during D-periods. Aside from this, however, resting muscle potential, especially in the large antigravity muscles, is lower during S than during waking; but it is lower still, almost nonexistent, during D-periods.[6] Some mammals, especially the ungulates, may obtain a considerable amount of S-sleep standing up, but the degree of muscular relaxation necessary for D-sleep requires them to lie down.

Arousal threshold in man increases with the changes from stage 1 to stage 4. However, it is relatively high during D, almost as high as during the deepest portions of S-sleep.[7] This situation is even clearer in other mammals; in the cat and rat, for instance, arousal threshold is distinctly higher during D than during S (Jouvet 1962; Dillon and Webb 1965). The maximal muscular relaxation and highest arousal threshold, at a time when by EEG criteria sleep appears to be light, have led to the name *paradoxical sleep.*

Mental activity during sleep has been studied in great detail (see Foulkes [1966] for a review). Practically all subjects studied not only have D-periods but report some kind of dream if awakened from a D-period in the laboratory. This is true whether or not they recall dreams at home. In very verbal subjects it is often possible to obtain some kind of report of mental activity during awakenings at almost any time during sleep. However, there are prominent differences depending on the time of awakening: Reports from the D-periods generally (in 60%–90% of the cases) produce perceptual "dreamlike" dream reports; the incidence of reports is increased if the awakening is sudden. Awakenings from S-periods produce considerably fewer reports (0%–55%, depending on how the questions were asked). There are also qualitative differences: S-sleep reports tend to be more "thoughtlike" or "secondary process"; and there is evidence

6. Jacobson, Kales, Lehman, and Hoedemacher 1964; Jouvet 1962.
7. Williams, Hammack, Daly, Dement, and Lubin 1964.

that more reports are obtained when awakenings are made more slowly, suggesting that to a certain extent S reports may refer to content during the process of awakening. To my mind the evidence suggests that the experience of dreaming *always* occurs during D-periods, although of course it is sometimes forgotten, and that this experience does not typically occur during S-sleep, although some form of continuing mental activity during synchronized sleep may well be present.

In this very brief delineation of typical sleep in man, several points stand out as surprisingly constant in normal subjects: There are always two states of sleep, S and D. S usually takes up about 75% of the night and D, 25%. The appearance of S precedes the appearance of D. Stages 3 and 4, the deep slow-wave portions of S-sleep, always occur predominantly early in the night or early during the sleep period. The length of the S-D cycle is almost always 90–110 minutes.

Phylogeny of Sleep

According to our behavioral definition of sleep, most vertebrates—certainly reptiles, birds, and mammals—may be said to have some form of sleep. In fish and amphibians, while periods of quiescence and somewhat increased arousal threshold are present, these are not so clearly demarcated from the remainder of the animals' life; and for these classes of vertebrates no distinguishing electrographic criteria of sleep have been reported. Reptiles show behavioral sleep and have slow frequencies in the cortex resembling mammalian S-sleep; in a few instances brief episodes of a state very much resembling D-sleep have been recorded as well (Tauber, Rojas-Ramirez, and Hernandez-Peon 1968). Birds have clear-cut periods of both S- and D-sleep, although the D-periods are generally very short and account for only 1%–5% of total sleep time. Only a few species of birds have been studied so far.[8]

8. Klein, Michel, and Jouvet 1964; Rojas-Ramirez and Tauber 1970.

Most mammals have clear-cut S- and D-sleep.[9] Both states are found even in the primitive mammalian species the opossum (Snyder 1964). However, it has been reported that D-sleep is absent in one very primitive mammal, the spiny anteater (Allison, Van Twyver, and Goff 1972). If indeed this mammal is found not to possess D-sleep, this could have important implications as to when the differentiation of the two states of sleep arose phylogenetically.

Within the class mammalia the two states of sleep have been studied in a wide variety of different species. No very obvious relationships emerge as yet in terms of the amount of S- or D-sleep. The "higher" mammals, such as monkeys and apes, do not clearly show either more or less sleep or more or less D-time than the "lower" forms. Within closely related species, for instance among the rodents, the animals which are usually preyed upon, such as the rabbit, have less D-time than the closely related but more predatory rat. To some extent this is true across many species of mammals—carnivores tend to have more D-time than herbivores, with the omnivores in between. This makes sense from the point of view of adaptation and selection, since the complete muscular relaxation of the D-state would make an animal especially vulnerable during this time, and long D-periods would be especially disadvantageous to herbivores and to prey animals.[10]

Although the amount of time spent in the states of sleep shows no very clear relationship among species, there is a very definite relationship between the basal metabolic rate of a species and the length of the S-D cycle (usually defined as the time from the end of one D-period to the end of the next) (Hartmann 1967). It can be seen from figure 3 that the smaller mammals with higher metabolic rates, such as the

9. There are too many references to be cited individually. See Freemon 1972 or Hartmann 1967.
10. These facts are opposite to what would be predicted by an "arousal" hypothesis of the functions of D; if D arouses or alerts the animals, prey species would benefit from more D-time or at least from more D-periods.

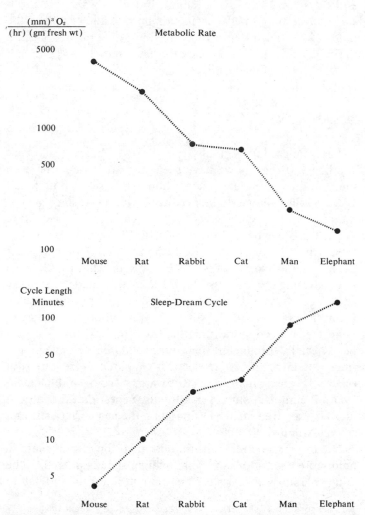

Figure 3. Basal metabolic rate and length of the sleep-dream cycle for six mammalian species. Reprinted from Hartmann (1967).

mouse, have shorter sleep-dream cycles and that an inverse relationship holds between the metabolic rate of the species and the sleep-dream cycle length. Indeed the same relationship can be found between metabolic rate and length of the pulse cycle, the respiratory cycle, the gestation period, and the life span. This establishes the fact that the sleep-dream cycle, also called the basic rest-activity cycle (Kleitman 1963), is indeed one of the basic cycles of the mammalian body.

Ontogeny of Sleep

The young adult generally spends 16–17 hours awake and 7–8 hours asleep. As we have seen, perhaps 6 hours of sleep time are spent in S-sleep and 1½ hours in D-sleep. Both S and D are on the average slightly reduced with increasing age, but the most striking changes occur very early in life (see figure 4).[11] Thus, a newborn child spends 16–18 hours asleep and at least half of his sleep is spent in the D-state. Although exact definition and scoring of S and D are somewhat problematic in very young children, this finding has been made repeatedly and suggests that D-sleep is an especially primitive state. From the point of view of function, it is important to keep in mind that if sleep has a functional role to play, this role may be especially prominent in young children and neonates, since at these times D-sleep is apparently required in especially great quantities (Roffwarg, Muzio, and Dement 1966). Preliminary studies in animals suggest that the fetus in utero has an even higher D-time than the newborn (Astic and Jouvet-Monnier 1970).

The ontogenetic relationship described for man appears to hold more or less for other mammalian species as well.[12] The young mammal always sleeps more than the adult and has an

11. Passouant, Cadilhac, Delange, Callamand, and Kasabgui 1964.
12. Cadilhac, Passouant-Fontaine, and Passouant 1962; Jouvet, Valatx, and Jouvet 1961; Meier and Berger 1965.

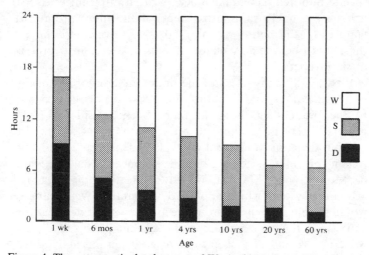

Figure 4. The ontogenetic development of W- (waking), S-, and D-states in man, in terms of the time spent in each state. Reprinted from Hartmann (1967).

especially high percentage of D-time. Also, the sleep-dream cycle, or basic rest-activity cycle, is clearly present at birth and is generally shorter in the newborn child or animal than in the adult of the same species. Thus the newborn human child spends his entire 24 hours cycling between W, S, and D, and the cycle length is 50–60 minutes. During the child's development the 60-minute cycle is gradually lengthened to 90 minutes, and a 24-hour sleep-wake cycle is superimposed upon it so that the adult pattern, in which there is usually one sleep period (occasionally two) during the 24 hours, is finally achieved.

Neurophysiology of Sleep

The exact neural mechanisms controlling sleep and its various states comprise an extremely complex field in which several hundred papers have been written in recent years.[13] I can only roughly summarize some of the more prominent features of the neurophysiology of sleep, concentrating on those that I believe may be useful to us in later considerations of sleep functions.

First of all, many areas of the brain, including parts of the cortex, thalamus, and hypothalamus, as well as large portions of the brain stem, have at times been considered sleep centers. There is, in fact, no question that portions of the midline thalamus and the hypothalamus play at least some role in controlling sleep. For a time it appeared that the work of Moruzzi and Magoun (1949) delineating the reticular activating system, which apparently maintained wakefulness, would simplify the problems of sleep. They suggested that the activity of the reticular activating system prevailed during wakefulness, and that sleep supervened when this activity fell below a certain level. This is known as the passive theory of sleep.

Recently, it has become obvious that this view is at best incomplete. In addition to the reticular activating system maintaining wakefulness, a number of brain-stem areas have been discovered to be involved in the production or maintenance of the two states of sleep. Thus brain transection and lesion studies have established an area in the medulla responsible for initiating S-sleep which actively inhibits the reticular activating system (Moruzzi 1962–63), and one or more areas in the pontine brain stem have been localized which are necessary for the appearance and maintenance of D-sleep (Jouvet 1961, 1962).

Physiological and neurophysiological studies have also suggested some subdivisions within S- and D-sleep. Recently the manifestations of the D-period have been divided into tonic and phasic components. The tonic components are those which persist throughout the D-period, for instance the dropout of muscle potential and the desynchronized activity

13. For reviews see Koella 1967; Hobson and McCarley 1971; Pompeiano 1970.

in the EEG. Phasic events include the rapid eye movements and other small-muscle twitches. The various peripheral phasic events have in recent years been related to central events, at least in the cat where all the phasic events have been found to be temporally closely related to a very prominent bursting spike activity found especially in the pons, the lateral geniculate body, and the occipital cortex.[14] These spikes have been known as PGO spikes and have played an important role in recent sleep research for several reasons: They occur at the very beginning of a D-period and sometimes herald its onset before the other signs appear; thus they may have something to do with the initiation of D-periods. Also, the density, or number of spikes per minute, seems to be some indication of need or "pressure" for D-periods; after D-deprivation, for instance, D-periods are characterized by a heavy concentration of PGO spikes. It was suggested at one time that whereas total sleep is only roughly recovered after deprivation, and D-sleep is recovered somewhat more precisely, the number of spikes is recovered almost exactly; however, this relationship does not appear to hold as well as was first thought. It has also been proposed that the spikes are somehow essential and must occur at one time or another; when they are kept from accompanying D-periods because of chemical or pathological situations, they will then occur at other times. It has further been suggested that schizophrenic hallucinations could be related to the occurrence of PGO spikes during wakefulness.[15]

In recent years studies of single units (neurons) have become possible, and these have contributed greatly to our knowledge of the neurophysiology of sleep (Evarts 1967; Pompeiano 1967). In looking for areas most centrally involved in initiating or controlling one or the other of the states of sleep, for instance, one can look at temporal

14. Brooks and Bizzi 1963; Dement 1970; Dement, Zarcone, Ferguson, Cohen, Pivik, and Barchas 1969.
15. Dement, Zarcone, Ferguson, Cohen, Pivik, and Barchas 1969.

relationships and examine where the neurons tend to fire first when the organism "switches" from one state to another. By such techniques McCarley and Hobson (1971) have suggested that neurons in the giganto-cellular tegmental fields are involved in initiating D-periods.

Such single-unit studies may also be important from the point of view of the functions of sleep. For instance, one possible hypothesis about function might be that cerebral neurons are resting and thus inactive during sleep. Based on studies so far, it can be said that this is not the case, or at least not the case for most of the large neurons studied up to now. (The fact that neurons with large cell bodies or large axons—generally Golgi type-1 neurons—are much more easily recorded from, produces some bias in the population studied; thus it is still possible that certain very small neurons may rest entirely during sleep.) Nonetheless, even though there is no cessation of activity during sleep, the firing patterns that have been found may be of importance for the functions of sleep. In many areas of the brain the general pattern found is that single neurons tend to reduce their activity during the transition from waking to S-sleep and then to increase their activity during D-sleep to a level as high or higher than that found during waking (reviewed in Hobson and McCarley 1971; McCarley and Hobson 1971). This, at the very least, suggests that active processes occur during D-sleep.

Chemistry of Sleep

Chemical views of sleep have been present in the scientific literature for many years. In one form these theories propose that there is a substance circulating in the blood, or perhaps in the spinal fluid, which is increased during wakefulness, especially during prolonged sleep deprivation, and which is metabolized or somehow disposed of during sleep. This was suggested, among others, by Piéron (1913) and Monnier and

Hösli (1964, 1965). Recently Pappenheimer has produced considerable solid evidence that there is a potent sleep-inducing substance, probably a polypeptide, in the spinal fluid of sleep-deprived goats, which is not present in the spinal fluid of control goats.[16]

In the recent past attention has focused more on brain chemistry and the contribution of certain chemical changes in the brain to sleep. A great many minor chemical differences between waking and sleeping in animal brains have been reported but cannot be reviewed in detail here. To my mind, one change that may be of importance from the functional point of view, and will be discussed later, is the finding of increased incorporation of phosphorus into brain tissue in sleep as opposed to waking (Reich, Driver, and Karnovsky 1967).

There is also much recent evidence that the biogenic amines—the indoleamines and catecholamines—are involved in sleep.[17] Reducing serotonin levels in the brain either by making lesions in serotonin-containing raphé neurons or by introducing a synthesis inhibitor, PCPA, greatly reduces total sleep.[18] In animals both phases of sleep are reduced approximately equally. Conversely, serotonin precursors can produce a reduced sleep latency followed by normal all-night EEG sleep.[19] Thus serotonin appears in some sense to control sleep as a whole, although others have suggested that rather than acting on sleep per se, serotonin controls the PGO spikes by maintaining them in their proper place during sleep.[20] The relationship of the catecholamines and sleep has been studied in detail and will be discussed in chapter 10.

16. Pappenheimer, Miller, and Goodrich 1967; Fencl, Koski, and Pappenheimer 1971.

17. For review see King 1972; Jouvet 1969; Hartmann 1970*b*.

18. Koella, Feldstein, and Czicman 1968; Mouret, Bobiller, and Jouvet 1967; Jouvet and Renault 1966.

19. Griffiths, Lester, Coulter, and Williams 1972; Hartmann 1971; Hartmann, Chung, and Chien 1971; Hartmann, Cravens, and List 1973.

20. Dement, Zarcone, Ferguson, Cohen, Pivik, and Barchas 1969.

Implications for Function

This is only a sketchy review of recent sleep research; a number of areas especially relevant to function will be discussed in detail later. This brief review may be useful, however, in our gradual approach to the functions of sleep: First, there are now certain broad well-established facts and relationships in sleep which must be encompassed by any theory of function. And, second, there are some striking findings, perhaps not yet broad or well established, which nonetheless demand attention because they point so definitely toward a particular hypothesis of function. As we have seen, some hypotheses as to function of sleep have been created solely to explain one or two of these striking findings. An adequate theory, however, should explain all of them, or at least point the way toward an eventual explanation.

To conclude this chapter I shall list the facts and findings which to my mind are especially important in these two senses and mention briefly the directions they suggest in looking for functions of sleep. First and perhaps most important is the existence of two distinct biological states of sleep in mammals. This fact must be accounted for by any theory and suggests that sleep may have two separable, yet related, functions. A theory should also attempt to make sense of the cyclical nature of sleep and the time intervals involved (although, as mentioned, this basic rest-activity cycle may have independent origins and be superimposed upon sleep). In chemical or physiological terms, such lengths of time would not characterize, for instance, conduction of nerve impulses, buildup of postsynaptic potentials, or most simple chemical reactions, all of which occur in much smaller time intervals. Minutes and hours would be more characteristic of processes such as transport of material within a neuron or synthesis of very large molecules.

A related fact to be accounted for is that under normal conditions S always precedes D and that in mammals with consolidated sleep patterns (such as human adults, who have

8 hours of almost constant sleep) deep slow-wave sleep (SWS) always occurs early in the sleep period. This implies that if there are two functions, one of S- and one of D-sleep, the S-function may precede the D-function. Thus one could postulate pairs of functions along several lines: *antithetical*— S produces, depletes, or alters something which is then disposed of, repleted, or changed back by D; in other words, D may function to "undo" some side effect of S's function (as in the reafferentation theories); *directly sequential*—for instance, S facilitates one chemical reaction, and D facilitates another one further along in the chain synthesizing some important molecule; or *indirectly sequential*—S is involved in synthesis or activation of a substance which is then transported, put in place, or used during D.

The phylogenetic data reviewed may also provide a hint as to function. The fact that the two states of sleep occur in practically all mammals and in birds implies that sleep is not required only by the "highest" or most specialized nervous systems. However, mammals do have a far more complex and especially more flexible and adaptive nervous system than other forms; and it is, of course, the growth of the cerebrum and cerebral cortex that makes much of the difference. Thus it would not be surprising if sleep played some role in maintaining the flexibility and adaptive quality of the central nervous system and especially of the forebrain. It may also be important that the two states of sleep are found only in homeothermic animals (birds and mammals), so that perhaps a relatively constant temperature is required for S and D to fill their roles properly.

The facts presented about the ontogeny of the sleep states suggest that whatever functional role sleep fills, it is required most in a very young animal. In terms of the quantitative shifts discussed, this statement would be even more true of D-sleep than of S-sleep. This obviously suggests that sleep might function in growth or maturation of the nervous system; however, we cannot be too specific, since a large number of tissues and organs show growth curves that could be compatible with the time curves for sleep as a whole, or for S- or D-sleep separately.

The prominent phasic events during D seem very central to the D-periods—it is these events, for instance, which become especially frequent on recovery from D-deprivation—and must be considered by any theory of the role of D-sleep. They do not yet provide any specific hints about function, except that the functions of D must allow for this pulsatile or sporadic character.

Another hint as to function comes from certain specific neurophysiological studies, which demonstrate that during D much of the forebrain is in a state similar to that of alert waking: the cortex shows desynchronized activity, blood flow is increased, there is a negative D-C potential shift (Kawamura and Sawyer 1964), and many species show prominent theta in the hippocampus.[21] The last finding has been associated with alert waking during learning situations (Adey 1966; Segal, Disterhoft, and Olds 1972) and during motor activity (Vander Wolf 1969). High levels of activity in the sensory cortex are also found during D (Evarts 1962), at a time when motor activity is strongly inhibited and sensory input is also greatly reduced or "occluded" (Pompeiano 1970). Thus the central portions of the sensory-processing-motor systems are strongly active, while their usual inputs and outputs are blocked. This obviously suggests active central (possibly cortical) processing, perhaps involving learning or memory.

Few chemical studies so far give any clear hints as to what chemical changes may occur during sleep. Reich, Geyer, and Karnovsky (1972) have recently shown that lactate and pyruvate levels differ somewhat in sleeping and waking, but the differences are not easy to interpret and depend, not only in magnitude but in direction as well, on whether the animal has adapted to the sleep situation or is sleeping in the

21. Cadilhac, Passouant-Fontaine, and Passouant 1961; Weiss and Roldan 1964.

laboratory for the first time. This illustrates the great difficulty in interpretation even of the small amount of data available. At the moment there is not a single chemical reaction in the body which we can say occurs only during sleep or only during waking; there are hardly any which we can say clearly occur more or less during sleep than during waking.

One chemical change that might point toward a functional role of sleep is the suggestion, not yet certain, of increased synthesis of at least some molecules or proteins during sleep (Shapot 1957; Reich, Driver, and Karnovsky 1967). Research has shown that there is an increase in incorporation of P-32 into brain tissue, most likely into phosphoproteins during sleep in rats. The time periods involved in these studies suggest that S-sleep is involved. Growth hormone secretion has been shown to have a clear peak in secretion during stage 3-4 sleep[22] and to shift with stage 3-4 when sleep is shifted to the daytime.[23] Taken together, all these findings suggest an anabolic, macromolecule synthesizing role, at least for S-sleep.

22. Takahashi, Kipnis, and Daughaday 1968; Sassin, Parker, Mace, Gotlin, Johnson, and Rossman 1969; Honda, Takahashi, Takahashi, Azumi, Irie, Sakuma, Tsushima, and Shizume 1969.
23. Sassin, Parker, Mace, Gotlin, Johnson, and Rossman 1969.

4 Sleep Deprivation

In medicine a classical technique for discovering the function of an organ is to remove it and observe what deficits follow. The analogous technique in sleep research is, of course, sleep deprivation, which by now has been the subject of many hundreds of investigations. Because of the findings reviewed in chapter 3, indicating that there are two distinct and different forms of sleep, I shall discuss here the effects not only of total sleep deprivation, but also of attempts to deprive a person or animal selectivity of D- or S-sleep.

The literature is profuse,[1] and the results of studies on sleep deprivation are surprisingly variant. I shall focus on two different sorts of effects of sleep deprivation—the physiological-chemical effects and the behavioral-psychological effects —but these are not always entirely separable.

Physiological-Chemical Effects

First of all, sleep deprivation if carried out long enough results in death. Animal studies have reported death in young dogs after 4 to 6 days of sleep deprivation, in adult dogs after about 13 days, and in rats and cats after similar periods (Kleitman 1963). There are many problems in these studies, including separation of sleep deprivation effects from other effects of the procedures used, but it seems reasonable that extremely prolonged sleep deprivation will result in death. During long periods of sleep deprivation common findings include a reduction in muscle tone, inability of the animal to maintain its normal posture, and a gradual fall in body temperature that occurs prominently late in sleep deprivation (Kleitman 1963). With shorter periods of sleep deprivation

1. For reviews of this area, see Kleitman 1963; Wilkinson 1965; Naitoh 1969; Williams, Lubin, and Goodnow 1959; Freemon 1972.

(1–5 days), results are not so clear-cut; Kleitman (1927), in a series of studies in dogs, reported no significant changes in heart rate or respiratory rate, in appearance of the blood cells, or in a number of blood chemicals. These studies found no neurological changes; however, a few other studies of animals reported certain pathological changes in the central nervous system, for instance in rabbits (Bast 1925). A number of chemical changes in blood and urine have also been reported (see Kleitman 1963; Wilkinson 1965; Freemon 1972 for reviews), but these results so far have not been entirely reproducible and do not fall into any obvious pattern.

Results in man show changes in the temperature curve, a gradual decrease in muscular strength, and a variety of inconsistent changes in blood chemistry. Again, large series of studies show either conflicting results or no clear changes in heart rate, blood pressure, basal metabolic rate, and the blood and urine chemical constituents for periods of 2 to 6 days of sleep deprivation.[2] In man there have also been a number of studies of EEG and other indicators of neurological function.[3] The EEG results show an overall tendency to lower frequencies and reduced alpha time, without much other change.

Overall, although sleep deprivation is obviously a stressful experience, and various autonomic and chemical changes that may be related to stress are sometimes found, there are few clearly demonstrated chemical-physiological changes produced by sleep deprivation. And, in fact, when such changes are found, it is not always easy to distinguish between the effects of sleep deprivation per se and the effects of the various techniques used for maintaining sleep depriva-

2. Kleitman 1963; Rakestraw and Whittier 1923; Kuhn, Brodan, Brodanova, and Friedman 1967; Kollar, Pasnau, Rubin, Naitoh, Slater, and Kales 1969; Kuhn, Meltzer, Wyatt, and Snyder 1970.
3. Blake and Gerard 1937; Tyler, Goodman, and Rothman 1947; Armington and Mitnick 1959; Kollar, Pasnau, Rubin, Naitoh, Slater, and Kales 1969; Johnson, Slye, and Dement 1965; Naitoh, Pasnau, and Kollar 1971; Naitoh, Kales, Kollar, Smith and Jacobson 1969.

tion—such as forcing the animal to walk slowly on a moving platform or a rotating drum.

However, there are a few hints relevant to function. Among the potentially important recent neurological findings is a significant reduction in *contingent negative variation* (CNV) after sleep deprivation (Naitoh, Johnson, and Lubin 1971). The CNV is an electrical potential from the scalp recorded only while the subject is waiting for an expected stimulus, and it is thought to reflect something like "attentiveness" or "expectancy" (Walter 1964; Tecce 1972). The results, therefore, suggest impairment in these functions after sleep deprivation.

There have been some attempts to summarize the physiology of sleep deprivation. Many authors speak of "reduced central arousal," while Ax and Luby, studying a variety of autonomic effects, summarize the effects of sleep deprivation more specifically as a "profound fatigue of central sympathetic centers" (1961). One of their striking findings was that certain autonomic responses not only gradually decreased but eventually reversed with increasing sleep deprivation—thus after 100 hours, diastolic blood pressure actually *fell* instead of rising in response to pain. Fatigue of central sympathetic centers after sleep deprivation suggests that sleep may have a function in restoring or maintaining central sympathetic systems. The ease with which centrally active sympathomimetic amines (e.g. dextroamphetamine) can temporarily reverse many effects of sleep deprivation lends support to these possibilities. For example, the CNV, lowered during sleep deprivation, is significantly increased by dextroamphetamine (Tecce 1972).

Behavioral-Psychological Effects

The behavioral effects of sleep deprivation have been studied very extensively in man, and there are some definite results in terms of deficits in performance.[4] However, one

4. Reviewed in Kleitman 1963; Freemon 1972; Wilkinson 1965; Naitoh

contradictory finding is the remarkable extent to which normal young subjects after days of sleep deprivation are able to "pull themselves together" and function entirely normally on almost all tests, or at least all tests lasting not more than 10 or 15 minutes. Performance on tasks requiring focused attention is often found to be impaired. For instance, recent studies by Hockey (1970) show a difficulty in the normal and optimal allocation of attention in a multicomponent task after sleep deprivation; in other words, it is hard for a subject to focus on one portion of a field and ignore other portions in a changing sequence.

Clearly, performance on a variety of tasks deteriorates after days of sleep deprivation, but there is also a strong motivational component, so that there is some question as to whether the subject is truly unable to perform a certain task or is merely less willing than usual to perform the work required. This probably accounts for the great variance in the results. Since most tasks suffer from sleep deprivation eventually, but since this is not very specific and may be influenced by motivation, it may be of interest to examine what tasks are most sensitive to sleep deprivation, that is, in which tasks are we best able to detect relatively small amounts of sleep deprivation.

A number of studies suggest that the most sensitive tasks are those in which prolonged concentrated attention or vigilance is required (Wilkinson 1964, 1965). Williams and his collaborators (1959) and Wilkinson (1965) have done extremely careful studies on sleep deprivation and its effects on behavioral and psychological measures. Williams et al. note that overall sleep deprivation reduces speed of performance on subject-paced tasks and increases errors on experimenter-paced tasks. Wilkinson has standardized different tasks, tested them on large numbers of subjects, and then listed these tasks in the order of sensitivity to sleep depriva-

---

1969; Williams, Lubin, and Goodnow 1959; Morgan, Brown, and Alluisi 1970.

tion (see table 1). As Wilkinson points out, the most sensitive tasks are those characterized by very low interest value, that is, extremely dull, repetitive tasks, and yet tasks requiring constant attentiveness. Table 1 refers only to a comparison of different tasks carried out for 20–30 minutes, but other work by Wilkinson (1964) makes it obvious that the length of the task is also important. Quite obviously, a long dull task will detect effects of sleep deprivation more than a short dull task. This can be carried to considerable extremes; for instance, Wilkinson has found that the only task capable of differentiating between a subject when he has had 8 hours of sleep and when he has had 4 hours of sleep is a task involving dull repetitive vigilance testing every other hour for 8 hours during the day (Wilkinson, Edwards, and Haines 1966). This is impressive, but it becomes obvious that the poor functioning of the sleep-deprived subjects may be a matter of literally being sleepy or even falling asleep momentarily while performing this painfully long and boring task. Also, factors such as motivation, anger at experimenters, and so on obviously become important. Attempts have been made to differentiate these effects from actual decreases in ability; for instance, Wilkinson (1970) suggests that subjects whose sleep was reduced to 3 hours per night had performance curves characteristic of lowered motivation, while only when sleep was reduced below 2–3 hours (i.e. when SWS was greatly curtailed) were there effects clearly related to decreased ability to perform.

There are numerous studies reporting effects of sleep deprivation on memory and learning functions. Again the studies are not consistent, but it is fairly clear that a word list, for example, which is learned in the evening will be better remembered the next morning if a night of sleep intervenes than if a night of wakefulness intervenes. This, however, is probably more related to the well-known effect of *retroactive inhibition* during waking—interference with memory by subsequent stimuli—rather than anything related specifically to sleep.

Table 1. Effects of Sleep Deprivation

Test	Level of Performance without Sleep
Serial reaction (gaps)	7
Vigilance (signals seen) whole test	34
Vigilance (signals seen) last half of test	4
Coded decision taking (errors)	45
Serial reaction (errors)	47
Chess	51
Card sorting (errors)	60
Card sorting (speed)	76
Serial reaction (correct responses)	77
Darts	97
Rote learning (errors)	100
Table tennis	100
Tactical decision taking (errors)	100

NOTE: The effect of up to 60 hrs sleep deprivation on various tests and scored games, all of 20–30 mins duration (level of performance without sleep is expressed as a percentage of the control level of performance with normal sleep). Reprinted from Wilkinson (1965).

On other scales and psychological tests it becomes obvious that subjects sometimes suffer from a wide variety of disturbances after sleep deprivation including illusions and sometimes visual and auditory hallucinations as well as inability to maintain a straight line of thought, loosening of associations, and some loosening of their usual ego defensive mechanisms. However, these findings are harder to quantitate and usually show up in a significant degree only after 4 or more days of deprivation.[5] On a subjective and less easy-to-define level, it is almost always noted that sleep-deprived subjects become increasingly angry, irritable, unfocused, and antisocial.

Trying to summarize all these behavioral and psychological effects of sleep deprivation is somewhat disappointing. For one thing, the poor performance shown on many of the tests

5. Tyler 1955; West, Janszen, Lester, and Cornelisoon 1962; Bliss, Clark, and West 1959.

can be explained simply by very short episodes of sleep ("microsleep") occurring in the sleep-deprived subjects; and just such episodes can be found on EEG recordings (Webb 1962). Thus, one well-known sleep researcher is able to state, without unusual cynicism, that after a long review of the entire sleep deprivation literature he has concluded that "the effect of sleep deprivation is to make the subject fall asleep" (Webb 1971). Without going quite to this extreme, we can agree to some extent that studies of sleep deprivation have been disappointing. I do not believe, however, that the very obvious subjective and emotional effects of sleep deprivation should be neglected, although these are more difficult to measure. I believe we are in one of those situations where we must carefully differentiate between problematic or fuzzy data resulting from the absence of any effect to be measured and problematic or fuzzy data resulting from our inability to measure properly an effect which is present. Obviously my prejudice is toward believing the latter. Yet, in summarizing effects on behavior and psychology, I will have to be satisfied with a general impression that after sleep deprivation the greatest difficulties are found in focused and prolonged attention and especially in focusing on one thing while avoiding distracting stimuli. Eventually, there is also a change in the direction of breakdown of normal ego defensive mechanisms, allowing the emergence of more primitive, usually repressed, material.

Recovery Sleep

So far we have concentrated on the effects of total sleep deprivation upon various aspects of waking which should be the most relevant in assessing the functions of sleep. One other facet of sleep deprivation that may be important is the study of recovery sleep after a period of sleep deprivation, and work in this area does show fairly definite and consistent results. Sleep time after periods of sleep deprivation is obviously prolonged over the subject's normal sleep time but is much less than the amount he would need to "catch up"; that is, after 3–4 days of sleep deprivation, a typical young subject sleeps approximately 12–14 hours and may sleep an hour longer than usual on the next night but not much more than that (Kleitman 1963). EEG recordings show that the first recovery night is characterized by high levels of stage-3 and especially stage-4 sleep, whereas in the second and third nights of recovery, or sometimes later in the first night, there is a great increase in D-time.[6] This suggests that deep slow-wave sleep and D-sleep are probably the most important portions of sleep, since the body "wants" these most; the studies further suggest that between these two there is a primacy for deep slow-wave sleep (SWS). Slow-wave sleep is indeed recovered first, but it always occurs first during the night, so the "primacy" may be a matter of temporal precedence rather than "importance"; slow-wave sleep may fulfill some function which has to precede the functions of D.

Selective Deprivation of S- and D-Sleep

It has recently become possible to a certain extent to deprive humans and animals selectively of the two states of sleep. There has been very little work on S-deprivation, since in both animals and humans it is impossible to produce complete deprivation of S-sleep leaving only D—any attempt at this produces total sleep deprivation. However, a technique has been developed in which stage 4, or the deep slow-wave portion of S, can be selectively removed without an excessive number of awakenings or a great reduction in total sleep time.[7] Studies using this technique demonstrate a recovery increase in stage 4 (Agnew, Webb, and Williams 1964) but no

6. Berger and Oswald 1962; Kales, Tan, Kollar, Naitoh, Preston, and Malmstrom 1970.

7. Whenever the sleeper's EEG record shows the onset of stage 4, a buzzer is turned on at a carefully chosen intensity insufficient to awaken him but sufficient to alter his sleep to stage 1 or stage 2.

clear behavioral results after up to 7 days of complete stage-4 deprivation on a number of physiological measures and behavioral tests (Agnew, Webb, and Williams 1967). However, the authors do note that the stage-4–deprived subjects tended to be physically lethargic and depressed, as opposed to the D-deprived subjects, who responded somewhat differently (see below). With this meager evidence one can only suggest tentatively that the functions of stage-4 or S-sleep may be to prevent, or to restore the body after, lethargy and physical fatigue.

D-deprivation is easier to achieve mechanically—it is possible to produce almost total suppression of D-time with very little effect on S—and, furthermore, there has been a great fascination with the idea of achieving "dream deprivation"; therefore, many studies on D-deprivation exist, both in animals and in man. Again, I cannot discuss here all aspects of D-deprivation, such as the rebound and recovery phenomena (see Dement 1970 and Freemon 1972 for reviews). Rather, I will restrict myself to discussing the effects of D-deprivation on waking behavior.

Several neurological effects are produced in animals by D-deprivation: Dewson, Dement, Wagener, and Nobel (1967) have noted a change in auditory evoked response, and several groups have reported a decreased convulsion threshold.[8]

Studies in animals suggest that D-deprivation produces interference with memory and learning in several senses. In experiments investigating the effects of D-deprivation on recall of previously learned material, results are mixed;[9] and even where effects of D-deprivation are found, alternate explanations are possible (Stern 1970). However, D-deprivation may well prevent normal consolidation of memories acquired prior to D-deprivation, so that the memories are

8. Ferguson and Dement 1967; Hartmann, Marcus, and Leinoff 1968.
9. Joy and Prinz 1969; Albert, Cicala, and Siegal 1970; Brill and Goodman 1969; Pearlman and Greenberg 1968; Stern 1969*a*; Leconte and Bloch 1970; Stern 1970.

disruptible, for instance, by electroconvulsive shock (Fishbein, McGaugh, and Swarz 1971; Fishbein 1971). There is also evidence that new learning is impaired by D-deprivation —in other words, that D-deprived animals will not learn a task as fast as will a normal or an equally stressed control animal (Stern 1969b; Hartmann and Stern 1972).

Since these studies have been performed almost exclusively in rats and mice, usually with fairly small numbers of animals, and there have been methodological problems (see below), the learning and memory deficits must be considered suggestive but not entirely proven. One study of D-deprivation in cats did show some learning problems, but basically few deficits were found; it was noted that the D-deprived cats are often hyperphagic and hypersexual (Dement 1965). A major problem in all these studies is finding adequate controls for various stressful and nonspecific aspects of the D-deprivation procedure. Another problem in evaluating effects of D-deprivation is that we cannot be certain from the usual deprivation procedures that all the characteristics of a D-period are actually eliminated. For instance, Fisher (1966) has shown that when D-deprivation in man is carried on in the usual way—by completely preventing stage-1 EEG associated with eye movements—penile erections are not totally eliminated, and erections which would normally only be found during D-periods occur during portions of S-sleep during the D-deprivation nights. Similarly, Dement, Ferguson, Cohen, and Barchas (1969) have found that after several days of D-deprivation, the important phasic PGO spikes begin to "escape" and appear during S-sleep and during waking. Continued D-deprivation, therefore, may not be deprivation of all aspects of the D-state.

Early studies of D-deprivation in man suggested that there were definite psychological effects of D-deprivation in the direction of irritability, suspiciousness, and possible psychosis.[10] More recent studies have found much less definite

10. Dement 1960, 1965; Sampson 1966; Dement, Henry, Cohen, and Ferguson 1967.

behavioral or psychological effects[11] and little or no effect on simple memory functions (Chernik 1972). One researcher (Vogel 1968) has concluded that REM-deprivation has no demonstrable detrimental side effects in man and that it can even help some patients with endogenous depressions (Vogel, Traub, Ben-Horin, and Meyers 1968).

Admitting that the evidence is so far not entirely persuasive,[12] there are nonetheless suggestions, in man as well as in animals, of interesting effects of D-deprivation. In some ways we can attempt to specify these more clearly in man because of the availability of interviews, mood scales, and other ways of obtaining subjective reports. Among the prominent but hard-to-quantify findings have been irritability, poor social presence, and defects or distortions of normal ego defensive functioning with at times an emergence of repressed impulses and conflicts.[13] In one study already mentioned (Agnew, Webb, and Williams 1967), the effects of D-deprivation and stage-4–deprivation were compared. Although significant differences could not be found on the psychological tests used, D-deprivation was noted to produce more difficulty in social interaction as opposed to the simple physical lethargy produced by stage-4–deprivation.

Recently, several authors have expressed doubt about D-deprivation results, and about the need for any D-time whatever, on the basis of studies indicating that some patients treated by monoamine oxidase (MAO) inhibitors over a

11. Kales, Hoedemaker, Jacobson, and Lichtenstein 1964; Vogel 1968; Vogel and Traub 1968.

12. Some researchers, however, look for changes after D-deprivation where no changes can be expected, i.e. changes in learning or cognition which are not found even after a similar number of nights of total sleep deprivation. Some critics have thus concluded from the frequently negative or indefinite results that D-deprivation has no effects; I believe this conclusion is not justified. It does seem, however, that too many small studies of D-deprivation have been done too soon. It would make more sense, perhaps, to establish clearly the effects of 5 days of total sleep deprivation, say, on measures of interest, and then also examine the effects of 5 days of D-deprivation, and/or stage-4 deprivation under similar conditions in the same subjects.

13. Greenberg, Pearlman, Fingar, Kantrowitz, and Kawliche 1970.

period of months had a D-time of zero or close to zero with little or no observable effects.[14] My own view is that reducing D-time by giving drugs which increase availability of catecholamines may not truly be "D-deprivation" even though D-time is reduced or even abolished. For one thing, in man it is almost impossible to produce mechanical D-deprivation by awakenings for more than 5–10 days, and yet it is amazingly easy to do so by using drugs; a different process seems to be involved. Also, in the rat certain learning deficits produced by D-deprivation can be reversed when one increases catecholamine levels by administering drugs such as the MAO inhibitors or l-DOPA (Hartmann and Stern 1972; and see chapter 10). All this suggests to me that these drugs do not deprive the organism of D in the same way that awakenings do; rather they may reduce D-time but provide a rough sort of substitute for D-time (although I do not believe that merely flooding the brain with chemicals can in the long run adequately fulfill the functions to be discussed for desynchronized sleep).

Implications for Function

From all these studies on deprivation, although many of them are inconclusive, I suggest tentatively that sleep may have a function in restoring the mechanisms of focused attention and possibly the mechanisms of learning or memory which are associated with attention. It may also function to preserve emotional integrity and social adaptation. All these seem to be especially functions of D-sleep. The view that sleep deprivation is a state of central sympathetic fatigue, the fact that many of its effects are temporarily reversible by amphetamines, and the finding that D-deprivation effects on learning can be reversed by increasing brain catecholamines all suggest the possibility that restoration of central catecholamine mechanisms may be a function of sleep and especially

14. Wyatt, Kupfer, Scott, Robinson, and Snyder 1969.

of D-sleep. This restoration could underlie the psychological functions of sleep, as will be discussed further. The only function suggested specifically for S-sleep is prevention of physical lethargy and fatigue.

It must be kept in mind that trying to find separate but related functions for S- and D-sleep, as we have done, is only one approach. It is also possible that all of sleep, despite the different EEG patterns and other characteristics of S and D, has a somewhat similar function. Thus, for instance, one recent study (Naitoh and Townsend 1970), has shown that after 2 days of total sleep deprivation, approximately equal restoration, as measured by a number of behavioral tests, was produced by 2 days of sleep from which D was selectively removed and an equal amount of sleep from which stage 4 was selectively removed.

5 Experiments in Nature: Long and Short Sleepers

Another approach to the question of the functions of sleep is to look at variations in sleep time found in nature and to try to relate this variability to behavioral or psychological differences. Thus, for instance, if one found that individuals who spend their days ascetically pursuing activity A manage to get along perfectly well on 2 hours of sleep per night, while individuals who indulge constantly in activity B require 16 hours of sleep per night to feel rested, this would give us a hint that we might look into activities A and B and investigate further anything in activity B which might require restoration by sleep. Life is, of course, not quite so simple; yet there are obviously considerable variations around the mean values of 7–8 hours of sleep per night obtained by most young adults, and it may be worth looking at what characterizes the life-styles or personalities of persons at the extremes of this distribution—"long" and "short" sleepers. Such studies can also be useful physiologically in helping to decide which portions of sleep may be the most essential. That is, if a person who sleeps only 5 hours per night nonetheless gets as many minutes of a certain portion of sleep as a normal sleeper, one might expect that this particular portion is in some ways essential.

In simplified form, the strategy of studying intersubject differences (long and short sleepers) pursued in this chapter and the strategy of studying intrasubject differences (variable sleepers) in the next chapter both aim at the same basic question: Are there situations characterized by an increased or decreased requirement for sleep? If so, how can we best characterize these situations, and can we then extract elements that might be studied more directly? The additional, physiological question is: When there is increased or decreased sleep requirement is the biologic structure of sleep altered, and if so, how? Answering this can clarify what

53

portions of sleep may be relatively invariant, or always preserved, and what portions change drastically with increased or decreased sleep requirement.

First we must ask, do we need sleep, and do we need a certain amount of sleep? Or do we merely sleep out of boredom or when there is nothing else to do or as an escape from waking life? Subjectively we certainly have the impression of requiring sleep, although the amounts we require and the times at which we require it may vary considerably. Persons who have tried to get along on less sleep than usual have sometimes found it possible to reduce sleep to 6, 5, or even 4 hours for a certain length of time, but seldom for long and seldom to levels below these.

It is also a fact that overall sleep time varies remarkably little as a function of latitude, climate, hours chosen for sleep, and societal patterns. Young adults generally tend to sleep 7 to 8 hours per night despite the greatest variation in all these factors. Kleitman and his collaborators found that even a most extreme change, that which occurs between summer and winter in northern Norway (midnight sun versus noon moon), is associated with only a small change in sleep time—50 minutes more sleep per night reported in the winter than in the summer (Kleitman and Kleitman 1953). Another study of men living in the arctic found even less difference (Lewis and Masterton 1957). This universal tendency to obtain a certain amount of sleep strongly suggests that in a mammalian species such as man, who is reasonably well adapted biologically to life on earth, there is some justification for these 7 or 8 hours spent sleeping, that they are not a temporal vermiform appendix that has outlived whatever usefulness it might once have had.

Studies of sleep deprivation also indicate that sleep is required—that the body suffers when deprived of sleep and makes an attempt at restitution—although these studies do not give a good quantitative estimate of requirement. The various studies of D-deprivation and stage-4-deprivation do suggest that homeostatic mechanisms are in effect to hold levels of these stages more or less constant and close to their usual levels.

In humans it is very hard to study sleep requirement exactly, since there might in fact be several different levels of requirement. For each person there could theoretically be an absolute minimum below which he is unable to live; perhaps another level below which he can remain physically alive but cannot function anywhere near his normal capacity; then perhaps a third level, the amount he requires to function grossly as a normal human being though he may still not feel perfectly well; and still a fourth level, what he himself would describe as his sleep requirement—the amount of sleep he needs to feel "himself," to feel well. We cannot of course differentiate clearly between these, but in studies of human sleep requirement based on instruments such as question-naires, we shall usually be talking about something close to the last of these -the apparent requirement which enables a person to feel the way he likes to feel, not merely to remain alive.

There is, of course, the additional question of whether a person really knows his sleep requirement; perhaps he is sleeping far more than he needs and would even feel better if he slept less. We have tentative data which suggest that this situation is relatively rare and that except for certain cases when a person may be escaping into sleep, the sleep he habitually gets and feels he needs may be considered a rough measure of his sleep requirement. A precise determination of sleep requirement, however, would require some kind of very sophisticated all-day testing of the person's usual complex functioning for many days, which is next to impossible and, if possible, would be extremely unpleasant for most subjects. (And the unpleasantness might in turn alter performance and perhaps even sleep requirement!)

Although sleep requirement obviously varies and may appear to be somewhat different depending on the exact definition, I feel that the general concept of sleep requirement is nonetheless a valid one, that many adults with stable sleep patterns can give a solid estimate of their sleep requirement, and that it is legitimate to discuss situations which may involve differences in sleep requirement.

My laboratory, in collaboration with Frederick Baekeland's laboratory in New York has completed a large-scale study of long and short sleepers.[1] Our subjects were selected and screened in a number of steps; at each step some subjects were eliminated from further study, but the data obtained were kept for evaluation. Notices were placed in daily newspapers in Boston and New York seeking males over 20 who always slept over 9 hours or always slept under 6 hours per 24 hours. The notice mentioned that subjects would be paid for participation in a medical study of sleep. Over 400 persons responded to the advertisements and called one of the two participating sleep laboratories. About one-third of these were eliminated during a telephone conversation on the basis of their having misunderstood the ad or having clearly irregular sleep patterns. A set of forms was then mailed to the remaining 260 subjects, consisting of the following: (1) a sleep log to be filled out daily for at least 2 weeks, which simply asked each day for the time the subject went to bed, the time he arose, estimated hours of sleep, any naps, and any dreams; (2) a sleep history form asking questions about habitual length of sleep, whether the subject ever needed to catch up on sleep, how long it took him to get to sleep and feel fully awake in the morning, and also asking questions about medical illness and the use of medications, alcohol, and drugs; (3) the Cornell Index, a form consisting of 101 simple questions about medical, psychosomatic, and psychiatric problems to be answered true or false; and (4) the Rotter Incomplete Sentences Test, a self-administered and easily scorable projective test.

At this stage, subjects were eliminated from further study under any of the following conditions: (1) if their home sleep

1. Hartmann, Baekeland, Zwilling, and Hoy 1971; Baekeland and Hartmann 1970, 1971; Hartmann, Baekeland, and Zwilling 1972.

Table 2. Sleep Patterns of Long, Short, and Normal Sleepers
Minutes Spent in Each Stage (Mean ± Standard Deviation)

Stage	Long Sleepers	Short Sleepers	Normal Sleepers
Awake	44.2 (±39.4)*·†	11.3 (±7.3)†	15.3 (±9.9)
Stage 1	17.3 (±16.0)	8.1 (±6.0)**	17.9 (±8.7)
Stage 2	261.4 (±73.7)†	167.2 (±15.7)**·‡	216.4 (±12.1)
Stage 3	22.5 (±8.6)**	25.0 (±10.0)*	34.3 (±13.8)
Stage 4	47.4 (±30.4)	53.3 (±19.5)	40.9 (±22.6)
SWS (3 + 4)	69.9 (±33.0)	78.3 (±23.9)	75.2 (±27.4)
D-state	121.2 (±35.5)*·‡	65.2 (±15.8)**·‡	99.7 (±29.4)
Total time after sleep onset	514.0 (±55.8)**·‡	330.1 (±27.7)**·‡	424.3 (±29.0)

* Significantly different from normal subjects, p < .05.
** Significantly different from normal subjects, p < .01.
 † A significant difference between long and short sleepers, p < .05.
 ‡ A significant difference between long and short sleepers, p < .01.

log showed a mean sleep time that was not under 6 or over 9 hours per day, or if 2 or more nights in 2 weeks did not fall into the indicated range (over 9 or under 6 hours); (2) if sleep history showed a marked variation in sleep times or a pattern of long or short sleep that had not persisted for at least 6 months; (3) if a serious medical or psychiatric illness was present; (4) or if they scored 8 or more on the Cornell Index or 130 or more on the Rotter test (either of which would suggest considerable pathology). Of 227 subjects who returned these forms, 52 were both accepted and actually appeared for further study.

These 52 subjects came to the laboratory and were given a brief psychiatric interview and took a Minnesota Multiphasic Personality Inventory (MMPI) test. Subjects were not studied further if they scored 2 standard deviations above normal on any MMPI scale except Mf (masculine-feminine). The psychiatric interview explored personality characteristics briefly and also investigated any areas that appeared problematic on the basis of the previous psychological tests. Thus, the typical sleep pattern was further clarified; some family sleep history was obtained; further drug history was obtained, as we wished laboratory study subjects to be as drug-free as possible; and the laboratory studies were explained to subjects so that any questions or fears about them could be discussed. Subjects were eliminated on the basis of the interview if they were judged to be psychotic, psychopathic, clearly unreliable, or if they were taking any drugs or medication except vitamins and occasional alcohol, nicotine, or marihuana.

After these procedures 40 subjects were accepted for laboratory study, and 29 actually appeared and completed the entire laboratory procedure. In addition to laboratory sleep, each of these 29 subjects were given another psychiatric interview and took the California Personality Inventory (CPI), a personality inventory similar to the MMPI but designed for normal subjects.

Each subject slept in the laboratory for 8 nights. The first 2 nights, spaced about 1 week apart, were considered adaptation nights. Nights 3, 4, 5, and 6, about 1 week after night 2, were consecutive nights in the laboratory. On nights 3, 4, and 5 subjects were given their usual indicated sleep time, but on night 6 they were allowed to sleep as long as they wished. Nights 7 and 8, spaced about 1 week apart, were dream recall nights on which the subject was awakened 5 minutes after the onset of his first D-period and 10 minutes after the onset of each subsequent D-period.

The physiological studies revealed some very definite findings. In tables 2 and 3 the data are presented as means and standard deviations for nights 3, 4, and 5 on all the young (age 20–35) long and short sleepers.[2] Data from nights 3, 4, and 5 for a group of average sleepers from another study in

2. Originally we hoped to study carefully long and short sleepers in various age groups; some of the psychological data covers subjects from 20 to 50. However, too few long sleepers over 35 could be followed through the entire laboratory studies to allow physiological comparisons in the 35–50 age group.

Table 3. Sleep Patterns of Long and Short Sleepers

(Mean ± Standard Deviation)

Stage	Long Sleepers	Short Sleepers
Number of awakenings per night surrounded by sleep	16.8 (±9.8)	12.9 (±11.8)
Sleep latency (minutes)	34.4 (±30.1)	17.1 (±19.1)
D-latency (minutes)	99.1 (±46.9)	93.8 (±18.8)
First cycle length (onset D_1 to onset D_2) (minutes)	107.8 (±23.4)	89.3 (±17.3)
Second cycle length (onset D_2 to onset D_3) (minutes)	122.7 (±19.0)*	93.9 (±11.6)*
Number of D-periods	4.5 (±0.9)*	3.2 (±0.8)*
Mean D-period length (minutes)	28.7 (±6.6)	22.6 (±6.2)
Mean REM density	0.179 (±0.083)**	0.114 (±0.054)**

NOTE: Data for comparison of normal sleepers are not available in this form.

* A significant difference between long and short sleepers, $p < .05$.

** A significant difference between long and short sleepers, $p < .01$.

our laboratory are included for comparison. The short sleepers averaged 5½ hours of sleep per night;[3] the long sleepers averaged slightly over 8 hours of EEG sleep, although they all spent at least 9 hours in bed. The most striking result in the study, clearly evident in figure 5 and in table 2, is that despite the great differences in total sleep time between long and short sleepers, they all spent almost identical and normal amounts of time in slow-wave sleep (SWS)—stages 3 and 4. Although the differences are not significant, the short sleepers actually spent several more minutes per night in slow-wave sleep than the long sleepers. Obviously the other portions of sleep make up the great

3. The results on night 6, as well as on certain vigilance tests, confirmed that the short sleepers were getting along on the amount of sleep they claimed and were not being sleep-deprived on nights 3, 4, and 5.

difference in total sleep between the long and short sleepers. The difference is especially marked in the time spent in the D-state—121 minutes in the long sleepers versus 65 minutes in the short sleepers (see figure 5). These values fall almost equidistantly on either side of the values for our normal sleepers. The long sleepers also spent more time in stage-2 sleep and more time awake. When these figures are expressed as percentages of total time, SWS of course occupies a significantly higher percentage of total time in the short sleepers than in the long sleepers, whereas percent of D-sleep does not differ greatly between the two groups.

The number of rapid eye movements per unit time (called REM density) is sometimes taken as a measure of the "intensity" of the D-periods. Situations such as recovery from D-deprivation are characterized by a high REM density, as are D-periods with reports of vivid, active dreams. The long sleepers actually had significantly greater REM density within D-periods than the short sleepers (see table 3). Thus the long sleepers cannot be said to have had long but less "intense" D-periods; if anything, their D-periods were even more intense than those of the short sleepers.[4]

Do the findings tell us anything about sleep requirement? On first glance, one might say that the long sleepers were simply poorer sleepers than the short sleepers. They spent more time awake during the night, had longer sleep latencies, and on interview generally reported that they did not feel as refreshed in the morning as the short sleepers. Are the long sleepers, then, well-compensated insomniacs—people who tend to sleep poorly in some ways but who are able to compensate for this inefficient sleep by remaining asleep for a long time?

In my opinion this is an insufficient explanation for the data. If our EEG tracings can give us any indication as to what may be important parts of sleep, we might look first at

---

4. REM density was higher in the long sleepers for each D-period of the night, as well as over the entire night.

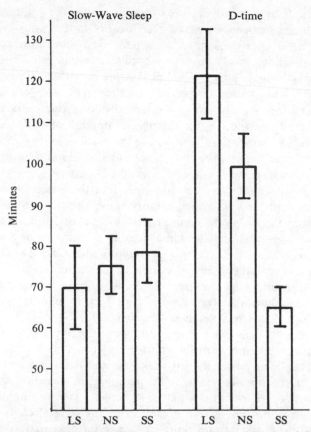

Slow-Wave Sleep   D-time

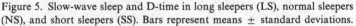

Figure 5. Slow-wave sleep and D-time in long sleepers (LS), normal sleepers (NS), and short sleepers (SS). Bars represent means ± standard deviations.

the deep, slow waves of stages 3 and 4, normally occurring within the first hours of sleep. The long sleepers obtained normal amounts of stages 3 and 4. If they are compensated insomniacs, unable to obtain these slow waves efficiently, we might expect the SWS to occur later or to be spread out over the entire night. However, this is not the case; the long sleepers concentrated their SWS early in the night as do normal and short sleepers. Then we might examine the

D-periods. A night of sleep is so arranged that the additional later hours of sleep provide a great deal of D-time; however, the long sleeper does not stop when he has accumulated a normal quota of D-time or of phasic events—his night contains roughly twice as much D-time and three times as many REMs within D-periods as the night of the short sleeper. This strongly suggests that the long sleeper is not inefficiently trying to get the usual amount of SWS and D-time, but rather that he is getting the usual amount of SWS but more D-time than short or normal sleepers and an even greater number of phasic events within D-periods.

In my opinion these results imply that there is a definite requirement for SWS which is fairly constant across subjects, since our three very different groups (long, short, and normal sleepers) all obtained the same number of minutes of SWS. On the other hand, if there is a requirement for D, as is suggested by other lines of evidence, the requirement is far from constant, and the great differences found between the long and short sleepers may be related to the psychological and behavioral findings discussed below.

Psychologically, we found a number of differences, on tests and interviews, between long and short sleepers (see table 4). Statistical analysis of the psychological test data showed that long sleepers scored in a more pathological direction than short sleepers on almost all test scales. The results that reached significance were higher scores by long sleepers on two of the Cornell Index Subscales—nervousness-anxiety and pathological mood—and on the Si (social introversion) scale of the MMPI; long sleepers received significantly lower scores on the L (lie) scale of the MMPI and on the CPI scales of social presence, tolerance, and flexibility. The following overall impressions from interviews and tests are based on the 40 subjects accepted for laboratory study, on whom the most complete data are available.

The short sleepers as a group were efficient, energetic, ambitious persons who tended to work hard and to keep busy. They were relatively sure of themselves, socially adept,

Table 4. Psychological Differences between Long and Short Sleepers

| | Mean Values | | Significance of Difference |
	Long	Short	
Sleep Log			
Home sleep time (hrs)	9.7	5.6	$p < .001$
Coefficient of variation of sleep time (hrs)	0.9	0.13	$p < .10$
Proportion of days with ≥ 1 dream reports	0.56	0.28	$p < .02$
Sleep Questionnaire			
Maximal length of sleep without interruption (hrs)	11.8	8.0	$p < .005$
Frequency of home dreams (per week)	2.8	1.7	$p < .05$
"Wake pill" (times taken)	0.57	1.62	$p < .05$
Cornell Medical Index Subscales			
Nervousness and anxiety	0.25	0.04	$p < .05$
Pathological mood and depression	0.42	0.09	$p < .10$
MMPI			
Lie scale (L)	2.8	5.2	$p < .05$
Social introversion scale (Si)	25.1	18.4	$p < .05$
*Interviews**			
When started sleeping unusual hours	ALR	AHS	$p < .005$
Positive attitude to sleep (negative, -10; positive, $+10$)	$+6.7$	-4.1	$p < .005$
Toleration of sleep loss (-10 to $+10$)	-3.3	$+5.9$	$p < .005$
Introversion (-10) to extroversion ($+10$)	-6.7	$+4.1$	$p < .05$
Overall energy level (-10 to $+10$)	$+0.8$	$+7.6$	$p < .05$
Aggressive drive (-10 to $+10$)	-5.8	$+0.5$	$p < .05$
Ambition (-10 to $+10$)	-6.7	$+3.2$	$p < .005$
CPI			
Social presence	57.6	64.7	$p < .05$
Tolerance	48.5	54.6	$p < .10$
Flexibility	53.2	61.3	$p < .10$
Mood-Adjective Checklist (on awakening)			
Overall			
Depression	1.6	1.3	$p < .10$
Distrust	2.25	1.40	$p < .10$

Table 4 (continued)

| | Mean Values | | Significance |
	Long	Short	of Difference
After first awakening			
Distrust	3.23	1.81	p < .10
Quiet	4.50	3.17	p < .10
Detached	3.91	2.44	p < .10
Changes during the night			
Increasingly active	0.89	0.02	p < .005
Laboratory Dreams			
Mean primary process score (Auld			
Scale)	1.86	1.36	p < .05

* ALR, "as long as I can remember"; AHS, "after high school." These represent the median and the mode; results could not readily be quantified. The other interview items were very roughly quantified on a scale of -10 to $+10$ by a rater who read the interviews without knowing anything about the subjects. Adjective checklist scores are a simple sum of points scored for each adjective belonging in a given scale.

decisive, and were satisfied with themselves and their lives. They had few complaints either about the study, about their life situations, or about politics and the state of the world. Their social and political views were somewhat conformist, and they wished to appear very normal and "all-American." They were extroverted and definitely were not "worriers"; they seldom left themselves time to sit down and think about problems—in fact, several of them, on being asked what they did in times of stress or worry, made statements such as "I never let my worries go to my head." They seemed relatively free from psychopathology; but insofar as there was pathology, it consisted of a tendency to avoid problems by keeping busy and by denial, which in some cases approached hypomania.

The long sleepers were a less easily definable group than the short sleepers. They worked at a large range of employments; several of them were "eternal students"; and they tended to be nonconformist and critical in their social and political views. The long sleepers were more uncomfortable in many ways than the short sleepers; they complained of a variety of minor aches and pains and also complained about the laboratory. Although none of them were seriously ill psychiatrically, most had mild or moderate neurotic problems. Some were overtly anxious, some showed considerable inhibition in aggressive and sexual functioning, and some were mildly depressed. They appeared, in general, not very sure of themselves, their career choices, or their life-styles; however, several appeared to be artistic and creative persons. A few were aware that they sometimes used sleep as an escape when reality was unpleasant. Most of them valued sleep highly and felt it important to obtain the proper amount of sleep every night. Overall, they were definitely "worriers" who did let their problems "go to their heads" and spent considerable time worrying over these problems. Likewise the long sleepers worried, or showed concern, about political and social issues far more than the short sleepers, who tended to shrug things off and not get involved. The long sleepers could be seen as constantly "reprogramming" themselves as opposed to the relatively "preprogrammed" short sleepers. Thus definite differences were found between the two groups; in a few words, the short sleepers tended to be "nonworriers" or "preprogrammed," while the long sleepers were "worriers" or "reprogrammers."

It should be mentioned that our results are not in agreement with one other, somewhat similar, study by Webb and Agnew (1970). These authors surveyed entering classes of college freshmen and chose for study those who claimed to sleep less than $5\frac{1}{2}$ hours or more than $9\frac{1}{2}$ hours per night regularly. They studied 22 short sleepers and 32 long sleepers, using psychological tests somewhat similar to the objective tests of our study, but no psychiatric interviews. Webb and Agnew reported no psychological differences between the groups, that is, they found only a few unrelated significant results, about the number expected by chance. In our study, however, this was not the case; out of 48 measures that could be considered psychological, 9 showed differences of at least $p < .05$ (one at $p < .005$), and an additional 4 showed differences at $p < .10$. Furthermore, the significant tests were in related areas and formed a pattern quite consistent with the more global impressions.

The different results can probably be accounted for by the difference in the populations studied. First of all, Webb's subjects were 17 to 18 while ours were over 20 years old; this in itself may make a difference, since we found on interview that sleep patterns often were not stabilized until age 17 to 20, especially in short sleepers. In addition, we found that among our applicants, aged 20 or over, college students seldom met our criteria because their sleep patterns were too irregular; most who thought of themselves as "short sleepers," for instance, reported sleeping only 5 hours per night for a few weeks but then sleeping very long hours one weekend, or possibly for an entire week after exams. Others reported napping in class during "5-hour sleep" periods. In such cases it is impossible to say whether the student actually had a low sleep requirement, and we would not accept him for the study. Therefore, it is probable that we were studying more extreme groups with more constant and established sleep patterns than those reported by Webb and Agnew. Our subjects had maintained their long or short sleep "style" for 1 to 20 years without change. Possibly some of the 17–18 year olds in Webb's sample were "experimenting" with styles of sleep which did not become their eventual life pattern.

Assuming that our results are valid, it must be kept in mind that we have established only a *correlation* between the amount of sleep and certain personality or life-style characteristics. I consider the most likely explanation to be that certain life-styles or certain personalities require more sleep than others. However, it is possible that the inverse relationship might be true, that sleeping different lengths of time could *produce* personality changes (for instance, some persons do report, at least over a short period, becoming slightly manic after sleep deprivation, and a recent study has found that depressed patients may, at least temporarily, improve after a night of total sleep deprivation [Pflug and Toelle 1971]). Another possible alternative is that there is *no* relationship—that both sleep time and personality are entirely independent effects of some third cause, possibly a genetic or early environmental factor. Evidence presented in the next chapter, on "variable" sleepers, will strongly support the first of these three logical possibilities.

If we assume for a moment that there is a relationship between personality and sleep time and that the "worrier" kind of persons require more sleep, it then appears probable from this study that they do *not* require more stage 3 and 4, but that they especially require increased D-time. Further, our study suggests that the long sleepers may have more "dreamlike" dreams and possibly make more use of their dreaming. Besides having far more D-time, the long sleepers have longer dream reports on laboratory awakenings (although the length of time before awakening is kept constant), and they have more primary process in their dreams (Hartmann, Baekeland, and Zwilling 1972). The long sleepers also remember more dreams at home under normal conditions than do the short sleepers. Furthermore, our relatively crude scales for affect on dream awakenings during the night showed a highly significant change across the night in long sleepers but not in short sleepers; long sleepers rated themselves as feeling more quiet and passive early in the night and more active and energetic on later awakenings, whereas the short sleepers had no change. Thus, the long sleepers appear to be experiencing some psychological changes during sleep, possibly related to their sleep patterns of high D-time and active dreams.

In addition, the simple physiological D-deprivation effect (i.e. subsequent D-periods come closer together—the cycle becomes shorter) was found much more prominently in long than in short sleepers after the partial D-deprivation produced by the awakenings during D-periods; the long sleepers seemed to be "trying harder" to have D-periods. In other words, there appears to be a quantitative difference such that the psychological restorative properties of sleep may be more important to some persons than to others, and reasonably enough it is the former who get more sleep (long sleepers). The possibility must also be considered, though it cannot be clarified at present, that there may be qualitative differences as well—that within a broad general function, sleep may actually serve different functions in different persons.

There are various bits of anecdotal evidence about long and short sleepers that may be relevant. Great men and geniuses are often reported to be either very long or very short sleepers. Edison and Napoleon are examples of persons who were reputed to get along on 4–6 hours of sleep per day regularly. Einstein was reported to be a very long sleeper. From a number of interviews, aside from the main study, I have gotten the impression that certain very creative, concerned persons both in art and in science often are long sleepers. One might suggest very roughly that great men in the sense of "tortured geniuses" might be more likely to be long sleepers,[5] while great men in the sense of extremely effective practical persons—administrators, applied scientists, political leaders perhaps—may tend to be short sleepers. This is based on very meager evidence, but it does fit roughly into the personality patterns found in our study.

One problem is whether we have studied true differences in sleep requirement or whether it is more a matter of persons training themselves to get along on varying amounts of sleep. Since there is no question that such training can occur, an extreme position might be that short sleepers are persons with great willpower who have been able to make themselves stop wasting time and have thus given themselves more time for activity, while long sleepers are self-indulgent types who do

5. Assuming that they do not become insomniacs, who then cannot be classified as to sleep requirement.

not have the requisite willpower. (I have indeed come across such opinions about sleep in interviews—more frequently, it need hardly be said, in interviews with short sleepers than with long sleepers!) It is of course true that there are great subjective elements in estimating requirement. Thus, on the basis of careful interviews and histories we chose long sleepers for our studies who always obtained more than 9 hours of sleep and who had attempted to get along on less but had done poorly and felt tired, irritable, and so on. However, we did not give them an extensive series of tests to see whether indeed they could have managed on less sleep, and in fact under circumstances which do not allow complete control of a subject's day, such testing is impossible. Even if one could somehow monitor behavior on various tests of function all day long, the factor of motivation would still be present, so that if inefficiency and poor functioning were found in such persons forced to get along on 8 hours of sleep, one might still say that it was not an inability to perform, but a lack of motivation. Thus, although there is no complete proof, my impression is that each person does have a rough sleep requirement, and this does vary between individuals; it is definitely possible, however, for someone to train himself to change within a range of perhaps 1 hour around his usual requirement.

Overall, these studies suggest that more sleep and more D-time are needed by persons with personalities or life-styles characterized by worry or by the dysphoric affects of depression and anxiety and by persons who tend to feel their problems rather than to push them aside. The long sleepers in some ways seemed more neurotic than the short sleepers, but they also included more nonconventional thinkers and perhaps more creative persons. The short sleepers were in a sense "preprogrammed"—functioning along smooth, previously laid down paths—whereas the long sleepers were engaged in worrying, new learning, and at times creating new pathways. Thus, longer sleep and more D-time may have some function in dealing with or restoring the brain and psyche after days of worry, depression, or disequilibrium or after difficult new learning—perhaps after any intrapsychic conflict. However, as mentioned, the cause-and-effect relationship is not yet clear and must await clarification by studies in the next chapter and eventually by direct experiment.

6 Experiments in Nature: Variable Sleepers

We shall now ask the same question as in the last chapter: Are there situations characterized by an increased or decreased sleep requirement? But here we shall seek our answers in changes *within* subjects rather than looking across groups of subjects.

I define *variable sleeper* simply as a person who has a stable enough sleep pattern and impression of his own usual sleep requirement so that he can note changes in it, and who does report times (lasting weeks at least) when his sleep requirement is altered. Variable sleepers, luckily, are much more common than long or short sleepers; thus we have not had to seek special groups, but have been able to send questionnaires to, and interview samples of, a normal adult population.

In the studies described in chapter 5 we have demonstrated psychological differences between long and short sleepers, and we have at least associated different personalities with different lengths of sleep; however, it must be kept in mind that we have recorded an *association,* but have not so far established a causal relationship. It may be that a certain personality or life-style requires more sleep; or, on the other hand, it may be that obtaining more sleep produces certain personality or life-style characteristics; or both could be completely independent effects of some third cause. A study of variable sleepers can help to differentiate between these possibilities, since we can examine behavioral-psychological changes and sleep changes in their natural time course.

We have completed two formal studies on variable sleepers and, in addition, I have interviewed a large number of variable sleepers more informally. The two studies each involved sending a questionnaire to a population of 1,000 to 2,000 persons. In the first study the population was equally

Table 5. Periods Associated with Increased or Decreased Sleep Need

	A Change in Occupation	Increased Physical Work or Exercise	Increased Mental Activity	Depressed or Upset Mood	Stressful Period	Times When Everything Going Well
Study 1 Reports of:						
Increased sleep need	42	81	57	71	60	9
Decreased sleep need	11	23	31	21	41	46
No definite change (or no such period)	190	139	155	151	142	188
Study 2 Reports of:						
Increased sleep need	29	83	67	81	69	4
Decreased sleep need	3	14	13	9	16	46
No definite change (or no such period)	226	161	178	168	173	208

distributed between faculty, staff, and students at a large urban university.[1] The second sample was chosen from voter registration lists in three urban and suburban communities (Brewer and Hartmann 1973).

After some preliminary questions about age, habitual sleep time, and so on, each subject was first asked to describe in his own words any period when his sleep requirement was greater or less than usual; then some specific periods or events were

1. Hartmann, Galginaitis, Moran, Owen, and Buchanan 1972.

listed (see table 5), and he was asked whether such periods or events had any effect on his sleep requirement. About one-third of the subjects who completed the questionnaires were further interviewed in person or by telephone so that we could clarify their answers and also gain further insight into the kinds of periods they were talking about. The problem that required most clarification involved a differentiation, when the subject indicated less sleep need under certain conditions, as to whether he really meant that he got along normally on a reduced amount of sleep, or whether he had misunderstood the question and was actually saying that he had difficulty sleeping—insomnia—at these times. In most cases we were able to make this differentiation quite accurately, and we kept only the answers of the subjects who clearly felt that their *sleep requirement* was decreased. (If the subject's answers, or the answers plus the interviews, made it clear that at certain times he slept less but that this was a matter of insomnia—inability to get the sleep he wanted—he was of course not considered to have a decreased requirement for sleep at such times, since his sleep requirement could not be estimated.) In the case of a report of *increased* sleep need, we had to exclude subjects who were merely saying they "got away from things" by spending a lot of time in bed (not necessarily sleeping). This line of demarcation was occasionally a thin one.

Between the two studies, a total of 501 usable responses were obtained; a summary of the results of the two studies is presented in table 5 and figure 6. On any given question a large proportion of normal individuals do not notice in themselves a clear difference in sleep requirement. However, 70% of the respondents noticed a change in sleep requirement under at least one of the conditions we specified. It is clear from the data that for most of those who did notice changes, sleep requirement increased at times associated with stress, depression, or change in occupation and at times characterized by increased mental, physical, or emotional work.

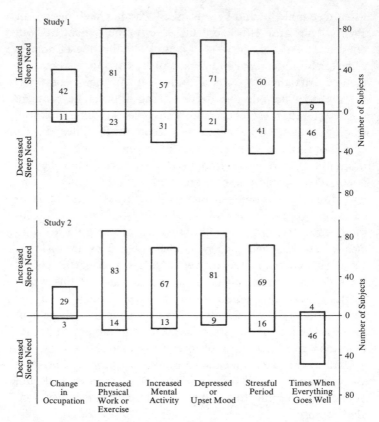

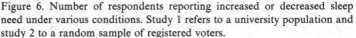

Figure 6. Number of respondents reporting increased or decreased sleep need under various conditions. Study 1 refers to a university population and study 2 to a random sample of registered voters.

Decreased sleep need was associated with "times when everything is going well" or involvement in work that the subject found pleasant. The changes in the direction of increased sleep with stress, change, or depression usually were found at times when there was a focus *inward,* on the self. An outward focus, on work, for instance, was often associated with decreased sleep need. Thus increased mental activity was usually related to increased sleep need, but a few persons clearly described *decreased* need at such times; it turned out they were speaking of pleasant and intensely involving work, such as "writing an interesting thesis."

The times when more sleep is needed, that is, times of stress, change in occupation, increased work, and so on, are of course overlapping and not independent factors; a factor analysis revealed one dominant factor dealing with stress, depression, and mental work.

The relationship of physical exercise or physical fitness to sleep may be a complex one. Although many subjects reported increased sleep need with increased physical activity, a number of very reliable introspective young men to whom physical fitness was important felt clearly that they required less sleep when they were in good shape physically and when they were obtaining an amount of exercise that made them feel comfortable. They needed more sleep when they did not obtain this exercise or were in bad shape or occasionally when they were physically overworked. Thus it is, in part, the factor of comfort and happiness—the egosyntonic quality of the exercise—that is important rather than the amount of physical activity.

Likewise, a number of persons with weight problems have clearly noted that when they are overeating and gaining weight or, for that matter, when they are trying hard to diet and lose weight, their sleep time is relatively long. They describe relatively less need for sleep at times when their weight is lower and more stable. Again, one factor may be that sleep time is less when they are doing and feeling well, when there is less tension and intrapsychic friction.

Aside from those noted above, there were a few other situations characterized by increased sleep need that emerged from the questionnaires and interviews. Prominent among these were pregnancy and physical illness; the first half of pregnancy especially was almost always associated with increased sleep need, as was illness when it was not accompanied by difficulty in getting to sleep.

These results within individuals are entirely consistent with those found across individuals in the study of long and short sleepers. Thus the majority of the variable sleepers had long sleep (experienced as increased requirement) at times when they underwent stress, when they worried and reprogrammed, or in other words when their lives were somewhat more like those of the long sleepers, and had short sleep (experienced as decreased requirement) when their lives were somewhat more like those of the short sleepers. Furthermore, the interviews often clarify the cause-and-effect relationship between lifestyle and sleep requirement in the variable sleepers. In certain cases it was quite obvious that an external event had occurred first—for instance, a death in the family, a loss of a boyfriend, a change in occupation—followed immediately by behavioral change, worry, or depression and subsequently by a change in the sleep pattern. In such cases it seems likely that the sleep patterns may have been caused by the changes in the life-style or mood; certainly the sleep changes did not cause the external events and closely associated activity or mood changes.

Not every variable sleeper responded in the same direction to the same situations, and it was possible statistically to pick out one or two somewhat deviant clusters or subgroups. There was at least one subgroup that seemed to be somewhat like the short sleepers, and this group sometimes showed changes in the opposite direction from the majority. When these persons felt stressed or upset, they responded by increased activity and felt that they required as little or even less sleep than usual. This appears entirely consistent with the "keeping busy" and "denying" personality characteristics which were found in the short sleepers.

In addition to the formal questionnaire study, I have interviewed over 200 patients and normal subjects about their sleep needs at different times. A number of persons have clearly described requiring more sleep and "wearing out faster" at times of depression and at times associated with stressful energy-consuming interaction with the world. Some saw sleep as also having a defensive function, helping them to get away from the world, but this was by no means always the case.

Five persons, all physicians, and none of whom expected the change, have described to me a considerable decrease in sleep requirement over the course of a successful psychoanalysis. They could not associate the change with any specific events in analysis, but it did seem to be related to a decrease of intrapsychic conflicts, less anxiety and worry, and in general feeling better about the world after treatment. This is certainly not universally the case, and it doubtless depends on the individual problems of the patient, but I have not heard any cases of change in the opposite direction.

A number of people involved in transcendental meditation have reported to me that their sleep requirement gradually decreased by 1–2 hours when they started meditating regularly. Again, this is not always the case and perhaps occurs predominantly in some individuals for whom transcendental meditation is successful in reducing stress and anxiety. On the basis of our results in long and short sleepers, we would predict that D-time especially should be reduced.

Many persons described definite changes in sleep requirement associated with changes in occupation and life-style. One especially striking case involves a student who had a marked change in his life about 2 years prior to the time of interview. He was a man in his thirties who had spent much of his life as a laborer. His typical day at that time involved moderately heavy physical work and very little thinking or worry. Two years before the interview, he had entered a distinguished university in a special program for intelligent persons who had not had the opportunity to attend college. His life changed greatly in that for the next 2 years he did chiefly intellectual rather than physical work; and, because of his limited previous schooling, slow reading speed, and so on, it was also necessarily a stressful and emotionally difficult time. He reports that his average sleep time has been 1–2 hours more in these last 2 years than previously and that he definitely requires (cannot get along without) this increased sleep. Again, increased sleep need is associated with intellectual and emotional work. I consider this case important because the sleep change was so clearly in the direction opposite to what would have been "convenient," that is, he would have loved to have slept less and to have had more rather than less time available for studying.

Several professional men, reliable and trained observers, reported that when they retired and stopped the considerable intellectual work and emotional stress that had characterized their working lives, their sleep requirement definitely decreased. Again, more sleep is associated with intellectual-emotional effort, and again the change is opposite to what one would expect (and they themselves had expected)—that retirement would be associated with more sleep.

I have spoken to 6 young women who clearly related periods of acutely increased sleep need to periods of loss— losing a boyfriend or parent or some other important emotional relationship. Here it was clear that the external event occurred first, followed immediately by some form of grief or emotional reaction, and followed subsequently by a sleep change over the next few weeks or months. This is important because here obviously the sleep change did not produce the external or behavioral change. A number of young women speak of increased need to sleep when involved in a "heavy scene" involving anger and depression. "At those times I get worn out and go to bed at 9 or 10 P.M., and I just can't quite wake up in the morning. I spend at least 10–12 hours a day in bed." Again, I have not spoken to anyone who reported a change in the opposite direction—requiring less sleep at such a time. People do sometimes report having difficulty getting to sleep or getting a good night's sleep at such times, but this clearly is not a matter of decreased sleep requirement.

Several combat officers have reported to me that in a situation in which soldiers were told several days before the fact that they were going into combat, the 2 or 3 intervening days were always associated with long sleep, often 12–16 hours per day. The officers felt that this happened spontaneously—the men seemed to get sleepy and need more sleep; it was not that the men planned to build up an "excess" of sleep in the expectation that they might not be getting much sleep in the days of combat. This situation seems to fit the pattern of increased sleep time at times of stress and worry.

The data reported here are based on personal interviews in a variety of situations which could introduce bias; nonetheless, I am struck with how consistently the results all point in the same direction, a direction very compatible with results found in the studies of long and short sleepers.

One extreme kind of variable sleeper, who will be discussed later, is the manic-depressive patient. My studies (1968a), as well as those of several other laboratories,[2] consistently show that at least among manic-depressive patients total sleep time is very low during manic periods and is surprisingly high during depressed periods—as high as or higher than during normal periods. The short sleep in mania appears to me to be a reduced requirement—when the manic period comes to an end, the patient does not generally have a huge increase in sleep which one might expect if there had been "sleep deprivation" for which compensation was required.

Concerning sleep in depression (see also chapter 7), it is obvious that some severe depressions are associated with disturbances in sleep (a large number of awakenings, etc.), in which case it is difficult to determine sleep need or requirement; but when there is no such sleep disturbance, sleep need appears to be increased during depressions. My view is that most or all depressions involve psychic pain and intrapsychic conflict which produces a need for increased sleep. But in addition to this some severely depressed or psychotically depressed patients have a sleep-waking difficulty which does not allow them to remain asleep for prolonged periods.

2. Platman and Fieve, unpublished studies and personal communication to the author; Detre, Himmelhoch, Swartzburg, Anderson, Byck, and Kupfer 1972.

Another situation relevant to variable sleep is the premenstrual period in some women. We have found that in detailed interviews at least half of all women describe some symptoms of depression, irritability, and so on in the week prior to menses. This is also a time associated with higher rates of suicide, homicide, and mental hospitalization than expected by chance.[3] At this time some women are also aware of a greater requirement for sleep. In the laboratory we found this late part of the cycle to be associated with significantly more D-time in certain women, especially those with the symptoms of premenstrual tension (Hartmann 1966a).[4] Total sleep was not significantly increased, but it was hard to increase total sleep under the laboratory conditions of that study. Several of the women reported that they did require more sleep during the week prior to menses and that they felt better if they allowed themselves to sleep longer at this time. This again suggests higher sleep need at times of stress or depression.

Overall, I believe that we can see a pattern of an increase in sleep need at times of stress, worry, defensive disequilibrium, and increased new learning;[5] all these can be seen as increased demands on the brain and the psychic apparatus. These results are easily reconcilable with the results of the study of long and short sleepers; and as mentioned, the

3. MacKinnon, MacKinnon, and Thomason 1959; Morton, Additon, Addison, Hunt, and Sullivan 1953.

4. This may not be the case in all women; a recent study (Ho 1972) of normal women without symptoms failed to find changes in D-time.

5. A fascinating question is how sleep, or increased sleep, fits into the person's own dynamics. For instance, falling asleep in the middle of a stressful or anxiety-provoking thought has obvious defensive functions, but this is not directly relevant here. Increased sleep at times of stress and depression likewise can be seen for some individuals as clearly defensive, as an "escape into sleep," while for others it appears merely as a "wearing out." The difference is very important in understanding the individual patient in psychotherapy, for instance, but I believe for our present purposes it is not essential. Increased sleep may well be required and may serve the same recuperative purpose whether the person sees himself as just tired out from a difficult situation or as specifically escaping from a difficult situation or, for that matter, even if he is entirely unaware of getting more sleep except in retrospect.

cause-and-effect relationship is more clear in studies of variable sleepers. Taking these studies together, I believe it would be fair to conclude that the first of the three alternatives mentioned in the last chapter is by far the most likely one—that certain life-styles or emotional states *produce* changes in sleep requirement.

Specifically, my conclusion would be that both across subjects and within subjects, worry, depression, certain kinds of stress, and increases in cognitive work and learning are associated with an increase in sleep requirement, whereas happy, effortless, "preprogrammed" functioning with a life-style of keeping busy and not worrying about problems are associated with a reduced requirement. Furthermore, the physiological studies suggest that D-sleep is the portion of sleep differentially involved, so that it is probably the requirement for D-sleep which changes under these different circumstances. In other words, these studies suggest that sleep has a function in processes of restoration after worry or stress, and perhaps after any waking "reprogramming" or "rearrangement." I shall try in later chapters to specify what brain systems may be involved in such restorative processes.

I consider these studies of long, short, and variable sleepers to be important evidence, though still of the "indirect," "experiment-in-nature" variety. There would be advantages to direct laboratory experiments in which some of the life-style and daytime activity variables are varied systematically and the effects on sleep studied. Such experiments are not easy to perform, but a few have been done and will be discussed in chapter 8.

7 Experiments in Nature: Age and Pathological States

Before going on to discuss the implications for function of direct experimental studies as to what factors can influence sleep (chapters 8, 9, and 10), we shall consider some further "experiments in nature" and examine how sleep is altered by age and by certain illnesses.

Age

Age is one of the few variables which show a clear-cut relationship to sleep patterns; the examination of this relationship may cast some light on the question of the functional role of sleep and the two states of sleep. In the newborn child total sleep time is extremely high—about 18 hours; it falls gradually to adult levels somewhere between age 10 to 20 and continues to decrease slightly throughout life. Even more dramatic is the decrease in D-time. In the newborn child D-time is 9 hours or 50% of total sleep. This decreases rapidly over the first years of life so that the percent is approximately normal (20%–25% of sleep) by age 5 or 6 though the absolute quantity continues to fall slightly (see figure 4).

There is relatively little change in sleep time between adolescence and old age, but the change that occurs is in the direction of a gradual, slight decrease in total sleep, in D-time, and in slow-wave sleep. The decrease in slow-wave sleep seems more dramatic, but this may be partly a matter of the definition of slow-wave sleep; the slow waves are still definitely present in older persons, but their amplitude becomes decreased so that less stage 3 and stage 4 is scored. The slight decrease rather than increase in average sleep time with advancing age does not seem to support Kleitman's notion of "wakefulness capacity." We would expect a biological "capacity" to be less present in old age and older persons thus to be less able to spend time awake; however, this is not the case. The data seem more compatible with the view we are developing that sleep may be connected with restoration after active mental or physical processes; since such processes occur less in old age, less sleep is required. The data could also be explained by the simple fact that sleep involves active neurophysiological processes which may diminish with age.

If the large amount of sleep early in life can be seen as a requirement (and it does seem very "necessary" both subjectively and as judged by behavior), one can then associate this long sleep with processes that are especially marked early in life. Certainly some of the characteristics we have described for long sleepers, or for variable sleepers when they need more sleep, are prominent in early childhood; it is obviously a time of intense new learning and reprogramming and usually a time of stress, worry, and intrapsychic friction (despite the lovely visions of carefree childhood we sometimes glimpse through our rose-colored retrospectoscopes).

Feinberg and others[1] have drawn a series of curves of various sleep variables over age (see figures 7, 8, and 9) and have tried to relate both total sleep and D-time to curves for oxygen consumption. The change in old persons with chronic brain syndrome (figure 10) is quite impressive: these patients have both a reduced cerebral oxygen consumption and reduced sleep time and D-time compared to age-matched controls. However, within the normal population the relationship between sleep time and oxygen consumption is less striking.

One can easily be misled by trying to generalize too much from the differences in shapes of age curves, especially considering that the scoring criteria developed for young adults may produce artifactual errors when used for other ages. Nonetheless, the impression that can be inferred from these age curves is that within the general decrease of sleep (total sleep, SWS, and D) with age, one can possibly

1. Feinberg 1968*a*; Feinberg and Carlson 1968; Feinberg and Evarts 1969*b*.

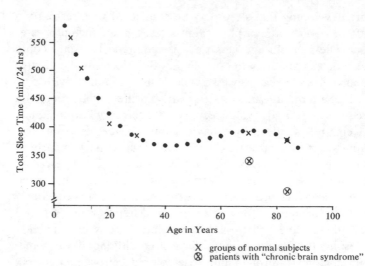

Figure 7. Total sleep time as a function of age. Reprinted from Feinberg and Carlson (1968).

distinguish two main types of curves. One is a simple hyperbolic decline with age—a rapid drop early in life and a gradual asymptotic fall thereafter; this is most characteristic of SWS and stage-4 sleep (see figure 9). The other sort of curve (cubic function) differs from the first chiefly in including a further sharper decrease in old age; this characterizes total sleep and D-time (see figures 7 and 8). Generally, it appears that total body functions, such as basal metabolic rate, follow the first pattern; whereas curves relating to the brain, such as total brain oxygen consumption, tend to follow the second pattern. This could lead tentatively to the conclusion that slow-wave sleep fulfills some requirement for the entire body, whereas D-time or perhaps total sleep time fulfills some requirement more specifically of the brain, and that total sleep, as we have seen in many different situations, is more closely related to total D-time than to total slow-wave sleep time.

Regardless of the shape of the curve, however, the early

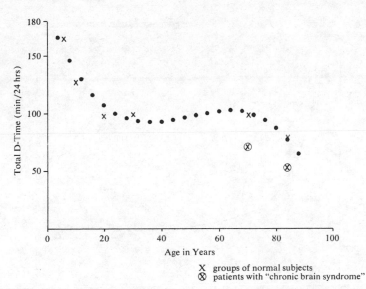

X   groups of normal subjects
⊗   patients with "chronic brain syndrome"

Figure 8. Total D-time as a function of age. Reprinted from Feinberg and Carlson (1968).

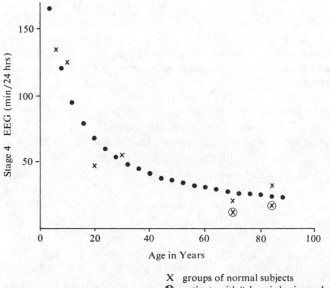

X   groups of normal subjects
⊗   patients with "chronic brain syndrome"

Figure 9. Stage 4 EEG as a function of age. Amount of change during maturity is appreciable. Reprinted from Feinberg and Carlson (1968).

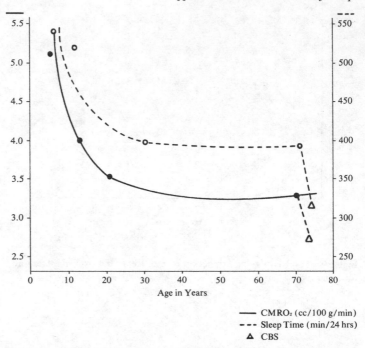

Figure 10. Cerebral metabolic rate (CMRO$_2$) and sleep time/24 hours in different age groups and in chronic brain syndrome (CBS). Reprinted from Feinberg et al. (1966).

rapid fall in sleep time and D-time are impressive, and they at least suggest that sleep has a function relating to some process that goes on to the greatest extent in childhood. Among the processes that come to mind are, of course, learning or organization of the central nervous system and also others such as growth of the entire body. The finding that certain groups of mentally deficient children have significantly less D-time than age-matched controls (Feinberg 1968*b*) adds weight to the view that it may be some aspect of learning or information processing, found to a lesser extent in the mentally deficient child, which is associated with high D-time in childhood. Along these lines D-time again might be seen as devoted to handling learned material or somehow restoring the brain after periods of intense learning.

Pathological States

Can the study of sleep in various pathological states help us in approaching the functions of sleep? I do not believe that a general survey of sleep and pathology is indicated; though, quite obviously, a variety of medical conditions can be associated with awakenings during the night and with disturbed sleep. This sort of association is important in clinical studies of insomnia and could be useful in helping delineate the neurophysiology of sleep control but cannot help us greatly in our search for functions. What could be important to us would be to identify pathological conditions in which requirement for sleep, or requirement for D or S separately, might be increased or decreased. If a decreased D-time is found, we shall again have to be careful, as in the studies involving long, short, and variable sleepers, to differentiate decreased sleep requirement, which would be of interest to us, from merely disturbed sleep.

It is widely believed, and this is confirmed by our questionnaires in the variable sleep study, that minor physical illnesses, such as colds or flus, are frequently associated with an increased requirement for sleep (Brewer and Hartmann 1973). This might suggest that more sleep, especially more slow-wave sleep, is required at times of tissue damage and that sleep perhaps plays a role in tissue regeneration.[2] This is supported by a finding that slow-wave sleep is increased in hyperthyroid patients (Dunleavy and Oswald 1972)[3] and is

2. In a preliminary series of studies on patients during the first days after a myocardial infarction, we have been surprised at the greatly increased total sleep time, but it is not yet clear what stages of sleep may be involved. Here again sleep could be considered a response to tissue damage or to the stress involved (Regestein and Hartmann 1972, unpublished studies).

3. Although one previous study showed no clear results (Passouant-Fontaine and Cadilhac 1966).

greatly decreased in hypothyroid patients,[4] who then show increases in SWS after thyroid administration. A preliminary study also has demonstrated increased slow-wave sleep in normal subjects on a starvation diet (Oswald 1972). These results strongly suggest that there may be some anabolic restoratory function for sleep, especially for slow-wave sleep. This is consistent with the finding (discussed in chapter 8) that exercise can produce an increase in slow-wave sleep. It may be that pain, or perhaps some neuroendocrinological changes set off by injury, are involved as well as actual tissue damage. For instance, Spitz et al. (1970) have found that S-sleep is greatly increased in newborn male children in the 24 hours just after circumcision. Here there is physical trauma, perhaps the first the child has experienced, but without any great tissue damage.

Some neurological conditions may be of interest in terms of total sleep and D-time. We have found that a group of patients with chronic Korsakoff's disease, which involves a defect in recent memory and very little ability for new learning, had slightly lower sleep time and, consistently, lower D-time than would be expected for their age.[5] Torda (1969) demonstrated lowered D-time in patients with recent encephalitis involving loss of recent memory. A very interesting finding by Greenberg and Dewan (1969) is that among aphasic patients, those whose aphasia was improving—those who were relearning—had significantly higher D-times than those aphasic patients who were not improving. These studies again suggest that D-sleep is increased when active learning processes are going on during waking.

As mentioned, total sleep time has been found to be reduced in children with certain mental deficiencies and in old persons with chronic brain syndrome, both compared to age-matched controls (Feinberg 1968a, 1968b). These studies showed that the difference was in both total sleep and D-time,

4. Kales, Heuser, Jacobson, Kales, Hanley, Zweizig, and Paulson 1967.
5. Greenberg, Mayer, Brook, Pearlman, and Hartmann 1968.

suggesting that mental functioning, or perhaps specifically learning ability, was related to D-time.

My impression from interviewing postlobotomy patients is that less sleep may be required after frontal lobotomy. One EEG study of this condition demonstrated changes in that direction, which however did not reach statistical significance.[6] If supported, such a finding might be important in that it would suggest more anatomic specificity: it would indicate that the waking processes we have been discussing—learning, stressful change, reprogramming, and so on—may involve the frontal lobes. A consistent psychological finding is that frontal lobotomy has often been noted to reduce excessive stressful worry in obsessional patients, for instance.

Can any relationships be found between psychiatric illnesses and the need for sleep? From the studies of long, short, and variable sleepers we found that conditions characterized by stress and anxiety were often associated with increased sleep time, but the subjects in those studies were among the so-called normal population. Can the same relationship be found among anxious, neurotic, or psychotic patients? Here the evidence is less clear. One obviously anxious group of acute schizophrenic patients had nights characterized by many awakenings, decreased sleep, and decreased D-time,[7] but other studies of schizophrenic patients gave mixed results. Likewise the first night in the laboratory, considered for most subjects to be a slightly anxious time, is characterized by somewhat low sleep and definitely low D-time. There are some results in the opposite direction, however. Rechtschaffen and Verdone (1964) found that relatively normal subjects who had scored high on the Taylor Manifest Anxiety scale had higher D-times. In a series of long-term studies on mental patients, we reported that times of psychic stress or disequilibrium and times of shifting defenses were associated

6. Jus, Jus, Villeneuve, Pires, Fortier, Lachance, and Villeneuve 1972.
7. Stern, Fram, Wyatt, Grinspoon, and Tursky 1969.

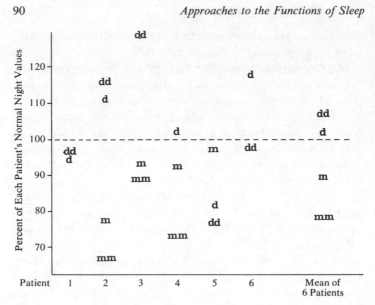

Figure 11. Total sleep time: summary of results in six manic-depressive patients. One hundred percent is the mean value for all nights rated clinically normal for the given patient; **mm** represents the mean value for all nights during manic periods; **m** is the mean value for all hypomanic periods; **d** for all nights during mildly depressed periods; and **dd** for all nights during severely depressed periods. The right-hand column indicates the mean of all the individual patient means. Reprinted from Hartmann (1968a).

with increased D-time and with decreased D-latency (time until the first D-period of the night) (Hartmann, Verdone, and Snyder 1966).

I believe the simplest explanation for these apparently contradictory findings is that there is a tendency for stress and anxiety to be followed by increased sleep and D-time, but that in some cases this is masked or even reversed by the difficulty in getting to sleep and remaining asleep when anxious. And disturbed sleep is almost always associated with a decreased percentage of D-time, since D-time is more sensitive than the remainder of sleep to noise or any physical disturbance. This is the same problem encountered in many interviews with variable sleepers: many had difficulty in getting to sleep at times of stress, making it hard to evaluate sleep requirement.

Depression and mania are known to be associated with changes in sleep. I have studied a group of manic-depressive patients in the sleep laboratory over a period of years. Results during manic periods were relatively clear-cut: mania was associated with greatly decreased sleep, averaging 4–5 hours, and D-time was decreased even as a percentage of this low sleep time; whereas slow-wave sleep was not greatly reduced (see figures 11 and 12) (Hartmann 1968*a*). In this sense the manic patients are extreme cases of the short sleepers; indeed, it was mentioned that there are also psychological similarities—the short sleepers tend to be somewhat hypomanic. The manic patient behaves in an exaggerated form of the style described for the short sleepers: he insists on being cheerful and not worrying, and he is preprogrammed, continuing to do things in his way while pushing away or denying painful realities around him.

Depression is more complicated. The textbook picture of a severely depressed patient involves disturbed and reduced sleep. Indeed, sleep laboratory studies of hospitalized depressed patients have generally found low total sleep, especially low SWS, and many awakenings—in other words, very poor sleep. Results on D-time have been mixed.[8] I have found hypersomnia in most neurotic or mild depressions and often in manic-depressive patients (see figure 11). My conclusion is that depression is usually characterized by a tendency toward requirement for more sleep and more D-time, consistent with an exaggeration of the findings in the long sleepers who, in fact, were often mildly depressed; in many depressed patients the hypersomnia and increased D-time can be demonstrated. However, I believe that in some severely depressed patients, perhaps especially in unipolar depressed patients, there is an

8. Mendels and Hawkins 1967; Oswald, Berger, Jaramillo, Keddie, Olley, and Plunkett 1963; Zung, Wilson, and Dodson 1964; Lowy, Cleghorn, and McClure 1971; Snyder 1969.

additional sleep-wake disturbance which makes it difficult for the patient to remain asleep. In such patients sleep and D-time may be reduced; but D-latency is very short and they have long, early D-periods, indicating that there is still somehow a requirement for more D-time than they are obtaining.

We have also demonstrated greatly increased sleep and D-time in a specific kind of depression, following acutely upon withdrawal of amphetamines. Here a great increase in sleep and D-time, and especially in REM density within D-periods, coincides closely with changes in clinical state (Watson, Hartmann, and Schildkraut 1972). This could be a special case because both the depression and the sleep changes may be produced by external chemical factors and may not be related to one another. Yet the temporal

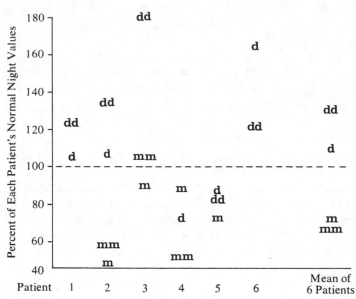

Figure 12. Total D-time. Summary of results in six manic-depressive patients. See legend of figure 11. Reprinted from Hartmann (1968*a*).

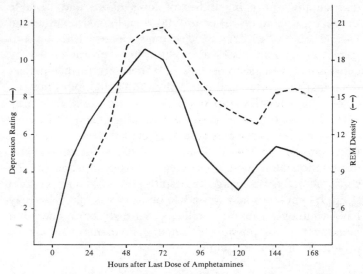

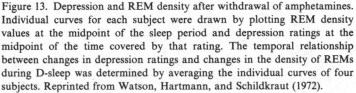

Figure 13. Depression and REM density after withdrawal of amphetamines. Individual curves for each subject were drawn by plotting REM density values at the midpoint of the sleep period and depression ratings at the midpoint of the time covered by that rating. The temporal relationship between changes in depression ratings and changes in the density of REMs during D-sleep was determined by averaging the individual curves of four subjects. Reprinted from Watson, Hartmann, and Schildkraut (1972).

correspondence of these two variables is striking (see figure 13).

Although premenstrual tension is not usually considered a psychiatric illness, in many women the week prior to menses is a time of increased irritability, anxiety, and depression. As mentioned, we found increases in D-time toward the end of the cycle in women with symptoms of premenstrual tension (Hartmann 1966*a*). Here again, increased D-time was found at a time of depression and anxiety.

The conclusions reached here from an examination of age changes and pathological conditions which affect total sleep and D-time are similar to and may amplify those we have reached previously in studies of long, short, and variable sleepers. In pathological conditions, too, long sleep and high D-time may be associated with times of new learning and memory formation and also with times characterized by depression and emotional "work." There are further indications that the cortex and especially the frontal lobes may be involved in these functions.

In this chapter we have also found some pathological conditions, involving tissue damage or increased catabolism, which produce increased slow-wave sleep as a response. This information, along with the decrease in SWS with age, but the constancy of SWS in adults despite great variation in total sleep, D-time, personality, and so on, suggests that SWS may have a biological function related to growth or regeneration of body tissues—possibly a function involving synthesis of protein or other macromolecules.

8 Sleep as a Response to Behavioral or Psychological Variables

In the next three chapters I shall discuss experimental studies in which psychological, physiological, and chemical stimuli are used as independent variables and sleep pattern is investigated as the dependent variable, or response.

There are, of course, any number of external stimuli which produce a change in sleep pattern in the sense of a sleep disturbance. This is interesting in terms of mechanisms maintaining sleep, and may be clinically relevant in studies of insomnia, but does not give much of a hint about functions of sleep, except perhaps that the lost sleep must to some extent be recovered. What is of interest to us here are stimuli—psychological, physiological, or chemical—which will produce as a response an increase or decrease in the *requirement* for sleep or the requirement for S- or D-sleep.

For this chapter our primary question will be: Are there behavioral-psychological variables which can produce such sleep changes as a response? This can be considered an extension of the studies of long, short, and variable sleepers; we can examine whether some of the same variables found in those studies to be correlated with increased or decreased sleep requirement, if now introduced as independent variables, will produce changes in sleep and the sleep states.

First, it must be said that it is not easy to alter sleep requirement by behavioral manipulations in the adult animal. Slow-wave sleep is especially hard to alter, and we have seen that it remains constant even under some very unusual total sleep conditions such as those found in long and short sleepers. The only behavioral manipulation which has been repeatedly shown to produce changes in slow-wave sleep is exercise: in man (Baekeland and Lasky 1966), in cats (Hobson 1968), and in rats[1] exercise will increase subsequent amount of slow-wave sleep. Sexual activity has also been

1. Matsumoto, Nishisho, Sudo, Sadahiro, and Miyoshi 1968.

reported to lead to increased slow-wave sleep in the male rat (Boland and Dewsbury 1971). A study in man involving comparisons of sleep after three types of evening activity also showed slightly more slow-wave sleep after the exercise condition, but results here did not reach statistical significance (Hauri 1968). Aside from this there are two recent studies, already mentioned, demonstrating that circumcision in the neonate (Spitz, Emde, and Metcalf 1970) and a starvation diet in normal adults (Oswald 1972) are followed by an increase in slow-wave sleep. This again suggests some metabolic bodily restorative function for SWS.

Many studies show alterations in total sleep and in D-time. Even some of the studies on exercise mentioned above throw light on D-time changes: in athletes accustomed to obtaining a great deal of exercise every day, a month without exercise was associated with only slightly reduced slow-wave sleep time but with an increase in D-time, and especially in REM density within D-periods (Baekeland 1970). Interview data make it likely that these changes were related to the uncomfortable and, for these athletes, quite stressful experience of going for a month without exercise.

If sleep requirement and requirement for D-time respond to changes in emotional or cognitive work, or stress, during the day, as we have suggested in the studies of long, short, and variable sleepers, is it possible to induce days of such conditions and study what kinds of sleep follow? A few studies of this kind exist in animals and in man.

First of all, both the kitten (McGinty 1969) and the young rat (Tagney 1972) in an "enriched environment," which allowed the animals great opportunity for interaction with the environment and for learning, showed more sleep and, in the cat, more D-time than matched control animals in an "impoverished environment." One recent study showed that rats have increased D-time during sleep after a maze-learning procedure (Lucero 1970). Leconte, Hennevin, and Bloch (1972) demonstrated a significant increase in D-time after avoidance-learning in the rat, and the amount of increase was related to the degree of learning. So there is at least some direct evidence that days of learning are followed by higher D-time.

In man there have been a number of studies in this area. One demonstrates that young adult subjects wearing inverting prisms (such that the entire world is seen upside down) have a very high D-time during the first days of exploring and adapting to this strange new environment (Zimmerman, Stoyva, and Metcalf 1969). Generally they again have high D-time when readapting to normal vision. There is still some question about these findings (Allen, Oswald, and Tagney 1971), but if true, they certainly suggest a role for D at times of cognitive reorganization and new learning. One study in which evening activity was systematically altered in balanced fashion between three conditions—chiefly exercise, chiefly studying, and simply relaxation—there were no significant changes; but the first D-period, the only one fully recorded, was somewhat longer in the studying situation than in either of the other two situations (Hauri 1968). Lewin and Gombosh (1972) have recently reported that when subjects are asked to spend 4 hours during the evening in a "perplexing atmosphere," in which they are asked to do a number of difficult and somewhat disturbing tasks without explanation, D-time during the night is significantly increased. This suggests a possible role in integrating emotional and cognitive data.

If indeed D-time is increased after days of psychic stress, disequilibrium, or intense new learning, and if this is a functional or adaptive increase, it should be possible to show that this D-time is useful, that the person is better adapted or working better the next day. Unfortunately, one great problem in both human and animal studies is the difficulty in evaluating adequate waking functioning. In animals researchers tend to be satisfied with observing gross behavior in an unspecified sense or, alternatively, training animals to do one simple task and then arbitrarily defining normal behavior as a normal number of responses on this particular task. In human studies the problem is even more difficult, since, as we have seen, a sleep-deprived person can usually pull himself together to function adequately at almost any brief task. On the other hand, trying to control the subject's entire day to check for various deficits or administering huge long-term vigilance tasks produces additional complicating factors: the subject's mood, for instance anxiety, or anger at the experimenter for torturing him in this way, and so on, obviously become increasingly important in the results obtained. In this context Wilkinson's studies (1966, 1970) are again relevant, since his experimental conditions involve a great deal of control over the subject's life. His results do suggest that at least 2–6 hours of sleep are needed for adequate function on his tasks, and he has inferred that SWS may be especially important for the basic ability to perform these tasks.

We all somehow assume that we function better after we have had a "good night's sleep," but there is little evidence correlating functioning in a more meaningful sense with subjective evaluation of a night's sleep or correlating subjective evaluation of a night's sleep with objective EEG criteria describing the night's sleep obtained. Still, it may be useful to inquire briefly whether obtaining different amounts of sleep or of its components influences how well one feels afterward. In one study of 110 nights of laboratory sleep in 12 normal male subjects under various conditions, there was a significant correlation between how well they reported feeling in the morning on a simple questionnaire and their amount of sleep during the night; there was also a correlation between how well they felt and the amount of D-time they had obtained (Hartmann 1970c). In a larger series, involving 711 nights,[2] there was a small but significant correlation between how well subjects felt in the morning and their D-time ($r = .173$, $p < .01$) but no correlation with SWS ($r = -.080$, N.S.) or with other stages of sleep. I have also studied a long series of naps in a single subject who filled out forms and rating

2. Subjects were taking either a placebo or one of five psychotropic drugs.

scales before and after each nap. The results were that naps with high D-time were associated with a decrease in "depression" and an increase in "energy" on a self-rating adjective check list. Also there was a high D-time during naps after which the subject indicated that she felt most refreshed or rested.

Greenberg and Pearlman (1972) have sought evidence for such a role in a long-term study of one psychoanalytic patient who sleeps in the laboratory once per month. Overall, the findings are that D-time is higher when there is evidence of stress or emergence of difficult problems (increased "defensive strain") the evening before the laboratory sleep night and evidence that these problems are improved ("defensive strain" is reduced) the next morning. Thus there is some evidence, though very meager at present, that increased D-time may fulfill an adaptive or restorative role.

Another important point has become increasingly clear as we integrate evidence from many different areas. This is that D-time and total sleep are closely related and change together, while SWS is harder to alter and is affected by a different set of variables. Thus, in the long and short sleepers total sleep and D-time were apparently correlated with mental or emotional factors, while SWS was invariant; human age curves for total sleep and D-time were similar, while SWS showed a different curve; psychiatric and pathological states produce similar effects on total sleep and on D-time; and the behavioral manipulations we have just discussed do so as well. The fact that total sleep and D-time seem to correlate much better than total sleep and SWS has also been shown in terms of correlation matrices in a large series of laboratory studies in normal subjects (r [sleep vs. D] = +.68, p < .001; r [sleep vs. SWS] = +.13, N.S.) (Hartmann and Cravens, to be published).

One explanation for these findings might be simply that SWS is more or less "completed" early in the night, while D is increasingly prominent later, so that whenever sleep time happens to increase, D is "passively" increased along with it.

There is some evidence for this in studies of extended sleep (Verdone 1968). However, in most of the studies cited here (long and short sleepers, inverted glasses, "perplexing" atmosphere, etc.) when D-time is increased, the increase is found even when measured in the first 6 hours of sleep, and REM density within D-periods is usually increased as well, so that a more probable explanation is that an increased "push" or requirement for D is primary, and sleep then extends to accommodate the increased D-time.

In this chapter we have reviewed studies attempting to alter sleep by direct experimental manipulation of behavioral variables. We have seen that SWS can be increased by exercise and possibly by sexual activity, by hypermetabolism, or by certain kinds of tissue damage. These findings again suggest an anabolic role for SWS. We have also noted that total sleep and D-time, which are often closely related, can be increased by enriching the environment or creating a situation of greatly increased learning, especially if it is mildly stressful or perplexing learning. This strengthens the hypothesis previously developed that D-sleep plays a restorative role in the brain, especially necessary when there is a great deal of new and difficult or stressful input to be handled.

9 Sleep as a Response to Physiological and Neurophysiological Variables

Here again we shall examine changes in sleep and in the states of sleep as dependent variables occurring as responses to other, independent variables; but we are now looking for independent variables in the physiological or neurophysiological realm. We are not interested here in the large literature on neurophysiological lesions, brain stimulations, and so on, which can disturb sleep or prevent sleep. Such studies are of course extremely important and give insights into pathways which may be involved in the production and maintenance of sleep or of wakefulness, but I do not consider them immediately relevant to the functions of sleep.

Are there physiological or neurophysiological manipulations which will produce as a response an increase or decrease in the requirement for sleep or for S- or D-sleep? Since a wide variety of agents or procedures can produce reduced sleep and reduced D-time, and it is often not easy to tell whether this is a reduced requirement or merely a disturbance in sleep, we shall be more impressed with independent variables or stimuli able to produce an increase in sleep or in one of the sleep states as a response.

First we will consider peripheral physiology and manipulation of steady-state environmental variables. It is not certain that any of these produce a clear change in sleep requirement, although many external manipulations produce disturbed sleep, usually characterized by decreased total sleep and especially decreased D-time. Such decreases have been reported with changes in external temperature in either direction, changes in barometric pressure, various illnesses and operations, and with a variety of noisy or disturbing nocturnal situations.[1] One exception that may be of importance is a

1. There are literally hundreds of studies demonstrating disturbed sleep and lowered D-time after chemical or physical interventions. For a partial

recent, not yet confirmed report by Valatx (1972) that maintaining rats at a high environmental temperature (35°C) produces a long-term increase in D-time. Previously, but under very different conditions, no clear change in D-time had been reported after high temperatures in the cat (Jouvet 1962). If true, this striking finding would support the role of sleep in restoration after hypermetabolism or tissue damage but would imply a special role for D rather than SWS in this process, as suggested by Oswald (1970).

Moving closer to the central nervous system, there are again a number of studies involving stimulation and lesions and their effects on sleep, but only a few are directed toward possibly finding a change in sleep requirement—that is, either a sustained increase in sleep or one of the sleep states or a long-term decrease that does not produce deprivation and catching up. In terms of stimulation, for instance, what we are looking for is not a stimulus somewhere which will quickly induce or interrupt sleep, but a situation in which a period of stimulation, for instance, will produce a clear increase or alteration in subsequent sleep or one of the sleep states in a repeatable manner.

One such study in cats by Frederickson and Hobson (1969) showed that 3 hours of powerful stimulation of the reticular activating system from a number of electrode placements produced significantly increased D-time during subsequent sleep. D-time was significantly increased for the entire 21 hours following the 3 hours of stimulation, though the increase was greatest in the first hours and D-latency was significantly reduced. Stern and Morgane (1971) have reported similar findings—increased D-time after intense stimulation of certain areas of the brain stem. This result, not very specific from the point of view of mechanisms or pathways, can be extremely important from the point of view of function. In Frederickson and Hobson's study D-time was

---

review see Hartmann (1967; in press); Hartmann and Wise (unpublished studies), and Kleitman 1963.

consistently increased after hours of nonspecific stimulation of a kind which is clearly arousing behaviorally[2] and produces a strongly aroused cortex. It is tempting to think that hours of such stimulation may be somehow similar to the situations we have described involving intense cognitive and emotional work or learning during the day. Indeed, situations of increased learning have classically been associated with cortical arousal. (I would speculate on the basis of indirect evidence, some of which will be reviewed later, that the ascending systems involved may include the catecholamine-containing medial forebrain bundle pathways.)

Adey, Bors, and Porter (1968) have demonstrated, in long-term polygraphic sleep studies of chronic patients with complete high cervical spinal lesions, a reduced D-time and a trend to reduced stage 4 as well. The latter can perhaps be related to the obviously decreased exercise and activity level in these patients. The former and more clear effect, the reduced D-time, may be related to the reduced input to the cortex, through indirect afferent systems (reticular formation) as well as direct afferents; in this sense the results support Frederickson and Hobson's (1969) results in the cat. Also consistent are results by Vital-Durand and Michel (1971) demonstrating a reduction in both D and SWS in "deafferented" cats, who have lesions blocking all major sensory pathways.

We have mentioned that after lobotomy in some human patients there may be a change in the direction of reduced sleep and D-time. A study by Villablanca (1972) showed that cats had a considerable and long-term reduction in total sleep and D-time after total decortication. The author interprets these results solely in terms of mechanisms producing sleep and suggests that pathways involving the cortex are probably involved in these mechanisms. From the point of view of

2. In this study the sites of stimulation were changed frequently to prevent adaptation, and the intensity was maintained at a level high enough to ensure constant behavioral alertness or arousal.

function these studies—along with those on lobotomy, high cervical lesions, and reticular stimulation—suggest that sleep and D-time may be high when a functioning cortex is present and obtaining high levels of stimulation from the brain stem during waking; while sleep and especially D-time are low in situations where this cortical activation during waking is not present. These results, of course, are entirely consistent with the high sleep and high D-time found in young children and the lower sleep and D-time found in some groups of mentally deficient children and in adults with chronic brain syndrome or presenile dementia. In this view the generally high D-time in children is not itself functioning as a "substitute" stimulation of the cortex so much as a restimulation, a reprogramming or restoration after the intense stimulation of waking life. There is probably a feedback mechanism sensing cortical activation and/or wear and tear and conveying the information to lower centers responsible for sleep and D-time.

In the last few chapters we have seen that the factors first noted in the studies of long, short, and variable sleep to be associated with increased sleep requirement—namely, stress, worry or depression, relearning, reprogramming during the day—are not merely *correlated* with longer sleep but can be introduced as independent variables which may *result* in increased sleep and increased D-time. And we have now been able to specify in a general way some neurophysiological inputs which produce the same results as stress, worry, and so on and may represent the central nervous system portions of the same inputs. In the next chapter we shall examine some biochemical characteristics of inputs or stimuli which produce increased sleep and D-time as a response.

10   Sleep as a Response to Chemical Variables

Sleep as a response can also be studied after chemical or pharmacological intervention. Again, many drugs produce merely disturbed sleep followed by subsequent recovery; this cannot tell us much about function. We shall be interested in chemicals which produce either a decreased need for sleep (or one of its major components) or an increase in sleep (or one of its major components).[1] When a drug decreases sleep, this more often appears to be sleep disturbance than decreased sleep requirement. However, there is one class of agents which may possibly produce a decreased need for total sleep in man: these are the monoamine oxidase (MAO) inhibitor group of antidepressants. One report states that 2 normal subjects taking MAO inhibitors for 6 weeks functioned well on considerably less sleep than usual (Kline 1958). My laboratory has conducted a small study using daily home sleep logs kept by the subjects. We found that three subjects who kept careful sleep logs over a period of 3 to 4 months, including 1 month during which either an MAO inhibitor (phenelzine) or the tricyclic antidepressant imipramine was substituted for placebo. All had significantly less total sleep (30–45 minutes less) during phenelzine or imipramine administration. No ill effects and definitely no feelings of tiredness or sleep deprivation were reported. These studies did not involve EEG recordings, but other studies of the effects of these drugs on sleep[2] make it extremely likely that it is D-time

1. One problem arises here which we have not considered before: If a chemical (drug) apparently increases sleep time, has an internal situation corresponding to an increased requirement for sleep been created, or is the drug having a direct toxic or anesthetic effect? The latter possibility is especially likely if sleep cycling and the natural sleep stage relationships are altered. I shall be careful not to consider the latter situation as increased sleep or sleep requirement.

2. Cramer and Kuhlo 1967; Jouvet, Vimont, and Delorme 1965; Wyatt, Kupfer, Scott, Robinson, and Snyder 1969; Hartmann 1969.

(and to some extent stage 2) rather than SWS which is reduced during these periods of antidepressant drug administration.[3]

Slow-wave sleep is hard to alter by drugs. In a large human drug study in our laboratory there was very little intrasubject or intersubject variation on stage-3 and -4 time compared to variation in D-time. This again corresponds to the findings in long and short sleepers. I know of no chemical manipulations which have been found to increase requirements for slow-wave sleep in normal subjects.[4] Some sleeping medications when first given appear to produce more slow waves, but there is a problem of whether this is an increase in normal sleep or whether the slow waves indicate mild anesthesia or coma. In recent studies some medications, especially the benzodiazepines, appear to produce a prolonged reduction in slow-wave sleep;[5] possibly this could be seen as a reduced requirement.

Drugs which Alter D-Time: Relationship to the Catecholamines

A number of pharmacological and chemical studies are relevant to producing changes in D-time. Most medications of various classes produce a slight decrease in D-time when first administered (Hartmann 1967; in press). However, there are certain medications which produce a very marked and striking decrease in D-time.[6] These are again the MAO

3. The MAO inhibitors, in which this effect on sleep is greatest, are now seldom used clinically. The more commonly used drugs, such as amitriptyline, do reduce D-time but have a perhaps independent soporific effect, so that total sleep is increased (Hartmann 1968b; Hartmann, Cravens, Auchincloss, Bernstein, Beroz, Marsden, Stanford, Sullivan, and Wise 1972).

4. However, sleeping medications or tranquilizers can sometimes increase slow-wave sleep in *insomniacs* whose sleep is disturbed and whose slow-wave sleep time is low.

5. Haider and Oswald 1971; Hartmann, 1968b; Hartmann, Cravens, Auchincloss, Bernstein, Beroz, et al. 1972. Kales, Allen, Scharf, and Kales 1970; Kales, Kales, Scharf, and Tan 1970.

6. And some studies report very little rebound increase after these drugs.

inhibitors and the other antidepressant medications.[7] Electro-convulsive shock in animals has been shown to have the same effect (Cohen and Dement 1966), and of course electroconvulsive therapy (ECT) is also an effective antidepressant. These treatments have another feature in common—they all make more norepinephrine available at central nervous system synapses.[8] This increased norepinephrine is thought also to occur in mania (Schildkraut, Schanberg, Breese, and Kopin 1967), which like the other conditions mentioned is associated with striking decreases in D-time (Hartmann 1968*a*). Likewise l-DOPA, a precursor of dopamine and norepinephrine, reduces D-time in the rat (Hartmann and Bridwell 1970) and, on intravenous administration, can "turn off" D-periods in man (Wyatt, Chase, Scott, and Snyder 1970).

However, as mentioned, it is relatively easy to disrupt D-time, and the opposite condition would be more convincing, that is, if decreased catecholamine levels produced an increase in D-time. We have conducted a number of studies indicating that this is the case. I reported some years ago that reserpine produces an increased D-time in man (Hartmann 1966*b*); it is almost the only pharmacological agent to do so. Reserpine reduces brain biogenic amine levels by interfering with their storage, but its effects are not specific to the catecholamines. It has also been found that in man methyldopa, a competitive inhibitor of dopa decarboxylase, produces an increased D-time for 2 days after a single dose, though the change is not large (Baekeland and Lundwall 1971).

We have recently shown that oral alpha-methylparatyrosine (AMPT), a specific inhibitor of catecholamine synthesis which lowers brain catecholamine levels by 50%–60%, produces a significant increase in D-time in the rat (Hartmann,

7. Akindele, Evans, and Oswald 1970; Hartmann 1968*b*, 1969; Wyatt, Kupfer, Scott, Robinson, and Snyder 1969; Zung 1969.
8. For reviews see Schildkraut and Kety 1967; Schildkraut, Schanberg, Breese, and Kopin 1967.

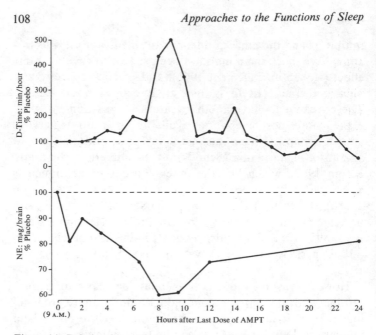

Figure 14. Relationship of D-time and norepinephrine (NE) over a 24-hour period after administration of AMPT, 75mg/kg orally. Each point represents experimental value as percent of placebo value; the curve for D-time has been "smoothed" in that the value plotted for a given hour is the mean of the previous hour, the hour indicated, and the following hour, e.g. the point at hour 5 is the mean of hours 4, 5, and 6. Reprinted from Hartmann, Bridwell, and Schildkraut (1971).

Bridwell, and Schildkraut 1971). This appears to hold immediately after a single dose as well as after long-term administration. Figure 14 shows results from our 24-hour studies of sleep patterns and brain norepinephrine levels studied hourly or every other hour after AMPT (75mg/kg orally in a single dose). This data shows that the greatest increase in D-time in treated animals, as compared to those given placebo, corresponded closely in time with the greatest decrease in brain norepinephrine levels.

Central catecholamine levels can be decreased in a completely different manner by administering intrathecal 6-hydroxydopamine which appears to produce degeneration of certain catecholamine-containing nerve endings;[9] after 6-hy-droxydopamine, brain norepinephrine levels remain low for months. We have shown that this treatment also produces a significant increase in D-time lasting at least 4 months (Hartmann, Chung, Draskoczy, and Schildkraut 1971) (see table 6).

This intrathecal administration of 6-hydroxydopamine also produced behavioral effects very similar to the effects of 3 or 4 days of D-deprivation: it reduced stimulation of motor activity by amphetamines, increased shock-induced aggression, and produced a trend to poorer acquisition of active avoidance-learning (Stern, Hartmann, Draskoczy, and Schildkraut 1972). In addition, when allowed to sleep, the animals treated with 6-hydroxydopamine showed a chronic increase in D-time, and this is obviously similar to what happens when D-deprived animals are allowed to sleep. Thus there are at least certain striking similarities between the D-deprived state and the state in which catecholamines have been reduced by certain specific chronic lesions of catechola-mine-containing systems.

These animal and human studies agree well with the effects of the antidepressant drugs and with the situation in mania and depression in man; it appears that conditions associated with high central catecholamine levels are characterized by low D-time, and conditions associated with low central catecholamine levels are characterized by high D-time (see table 7).[10]

We have also found this sort of relationship in several clinical studies of human depression. In a study of the depression following amphetamine withdrawal in addicts, we demonstrated a negative correlation, within patients, between 24-hour urinary excretion of MHPG (thought to be a good

9. Bloom, Algeri, Groppetti, Revuelta, and Costa 1969; Uretsky and Iversen 1969.

10. There are disagreements about some of these drug effects and the conclusions. For a review and a very different formulation see Jouvet 1969.

Table 6. Effects of 6-Hydroxydopamine on Sleep in the Rat

Treatment	No. of Animals	No. of 8 h Recordings	W-Time ($\frac{min}{\%}$)	S-Time ($\frac{min}{\%}$)	D-Time ($\frac{min}{\%}$)	No. of D-Periods	Length of D (min)	No. of Awakenings
Solvent	4	12	167.1 ± 17.5 / 34.6% ± 3.3%	266.0 ± 10.4 / 55.2% ± 7.7%	48.4 ± 6.4 / 10.1% ± 1.4%	24.4 ± 3.0	1.9 ± 0.04	37.8 ± 2.3
6-OHDA	7	19	143.1 ± 4.7 / 29.8% ± 1.0%	268.7 ± 5.9 / 55.8% ± 1.2%	69.7 ± 6.2† / 14.5% ± 1.0%	29.7 ± 1.3	2.4 ± 0.1‡	45.5 ± 2.2*

NOTE: W, Waking; S, synchronized sleep; D, desynchronized sleep. Values are given as means ± standard error of the mean. Values for W, S, and D under the horizontal lines are percentages of total recording time ± standard error of the mean.

* p < .05.
† p < .02.
‡ p < .005.

indicator of brain norepinephrine metabolism) and D-time measures (especially REM density in D-periods) in the following 24 hours (Watson, Hartmann, and Schildkraut 1972). In a study of hospitalized depressed patients we examined drug-free periods when sleep studies and urine collections were available and found a strong negative correlation, across patients, between MHPG excretion and D-time (Hartmann and Schildkraut 1973). Again, conditions where central catecholamine (and especially norepinephrine) activity can be presumed to be lower were characterized by higher D-time.[11]

Does this situation have any functional significance? I believe it does, but before answering this question we must consider the problem of what catecholamines or catecholamine-containing systems may be doing for the brain and for the organism.

Roles of the Catecholamines

There is evidence that the catecholamines are necessary for wakefulness. Jones (1969), in a study of midbrain lesions in the cat, has shown that both lesions of areas containing chiefly dopamine-containing cell bodies and lesions of areas containing norepinephrine-containing cell bodies can reduce wakefulness. Lesions of the dopamine-containing neurons reduced chiefly behavioral wakefulness, while lesions of the

11. I refer throughout this book to the catecholamines, since we have not been able to separate completely the effects of dopamine and norepinephrine. Both amines may be involved in waking (see below), but I believe the evidence overwhelmingly favors norepinephrine for the relationship with D-sleep I am discussing. The dorsal NE-bundle described by the Swedish workers (Anden, Dahlstrom, Fuxe, and Larsson 1965; Anden, Dahlstrom, Fuxe, Larsson, Olson, and Ungerstedt 1966) has exactly the properties required—ascending connections from brain stem to cortex and wide cortical distribution. In addition, the clinical studies referred to above showed highly significant correlations of D-time with MHPG, a metabolite of norepinephrine. Furthermore, we have shown that pimozide, a powerful central dopamine blocker, has no effect on D-time over a wide dose range (Hartmann, Zwilling, and Koski 1973).

norepinephrine-containing cell bodies produced chiefly deficits in the EEG signs of wakefulness—EEG desynchronization.

Table 7. Relationship between D-Sleep and Functionally Available
Brain Catecholamines

Condition	Catecholamines Available at Brain Synapses	D-Time (or D-Pressure)*
Imipramine	+	−
Amitriptyline	+	−
Monoamine oxidase inhibitors	+	−
Dextroamphetamine	+	−
Intrathecal injection of norepinephrine	+	−
Electroconvulsive shock	+	−
Clinical mania	+	−
Reserpine	−	+
Methyldopa	−	+
Alpha-methylparatyrosine (AMPT)	−	+
6-hydroxydopamine	−	+
Clinical endogenous depression	−	+
Withdrawal from amphetamines	−	+

NOTE: See text for details of some of these studies and for references.
* D-time changes in the direction indicated in all situations with the exception of some depressions. Here the situation is more complex (see text); some depressed patients show increased D-time, while others show decreased D-time, but with short D-latencies, long first D-periods, and high REM-density in D-periods, all usually interpreted to indicate increased "D-pressure" or "tendency toward D."

Several studies of intraventricular administration of small amounts of norepinephrine found behavioral activation and wakefulness.[12] We have found that intraventricular injections

12. Cordeau, De Champlain, and Jacks 1971; Segal and Mandell 1970; Hartmann, Zwilling, and Chung 1973. An older literature (reviewed in Cordeau, De Champlain, and Jacks 1971) spoke of intraventricular administration of catecholamines producing "sleep," but relatively huge doses were

of very small amounts (.01-30μg) of norepinephrine, almost in the physiological range, are able to increase EEG wakefulness and apparently also behavioral wakefulness (Hartmann, Zwilling, and Chung 1973). There is a good deal of indirect evidence that administration of l-DOPA, known to produce increases in brain dopamine but with relatively little increase in norepinephrine, has an arousing or an awakening effect in animals and in man. The amphetamines, thought to act by stimulating the release and preventing the reuptake of the catecholamines in the brain,[13] have classically been used in combating sleep deprivation and in increasing wakefulness or alertness. There is considerable evidence, then, that dopamine and norepinephrine are involved in the maintenance of wakefulness.[14]

In addition to this general maintenance of wakefulness, there is evidence suggesting some more specific functions for the catecholamines and especially norepinephrine during the waking state. Some of this must remain speculative, but I can briefly summarize my current impressions of catecholamine functioning during waking. (This has been reviewed elsewhere [Hartmann 1970] and will be discussed further in chapter 14.) The evidence is based chiefly on altering catecholamine levels by inhibitors of synthesis and by the effects of amphetamines, which, as mentioned, probably act by releasing naturally occurring catecholamines and diminishing their cellular reuptake.

One possible role of catecholamines, for which there is considerable evidence, is that active brain catecholamines at certain brain sites are involved in human mania and depression. Lowered catecholamine levels are thought to character-

---

used and there was little attempt to determine whether the state produced was physiological sleep, rather than coma, for instance.

13. Carr and Moore 1969; Glowinski and Axelrod 1965; Hanson 1967.

14. We are trying to differentiate further between these two amines by a number of means, but evidence does not yet allow us to say that one rather than the other is clearly involved in wakefulness. Quite possibly both play a role.

ize depression, while an increase of catecholamine levels counteracts depression (Schildkraut and Kety 1967). Human depressive illness is a very complex phenomenon, and it is my impression that the effects of raising catecholamine levels in depressed patients can be seen more specifically as reversing lethargy or increasing energetic behavior—this can be seen in animals as well as in human studies—and has something to do with increasing motivation as well as improving mood.

There is a good deal of evidence from inhibitor and releaser studies in animals that catecholamine levels positively influence motor behavior, usually studied in previously learned tasks.[15] Higher levels of catecholamines are associated with increased performance, and lower levels, with decreased performance. Human studies suggest that amphetamines and related compounds in some circumstances produce increased motor coordination and psychomotor performance (most easily seen after, but not restricted to, conditions of sleep deprivation or other states of reduced function) (Weiss and Laties 1962). Catecholamine levels also appear to facilitate new learning or short-term memory in a number of reward and avoidance tasks.[16] In one study catecholamine levels in two strains of mice were positively correlated with ability to learn avoidance tasks (Seiden and Peterson 1968). One review concludes with the statement that norepinephrine is probably involved especially in registration of information and short-term memory, as well as passage from short-term to long-term memory (Oliverio 1965).

The well-known effects of amphetamines make it probable that catecholamines are involved in functions such as vigilance or directed attention, as well as arousal or counteracting of fatigue (Weiss and Laties 1962; Seashore and Ivy 1953). These are clearly functions involving the reticular activating system. Some years ago Callaway and others

15. For reviews see Fuxe, Hokfelt, and Ungerstedt 1971; Hartmann 1970.
16. Doty and Doty 1966; Kulkarni 1968; Latz, Bain, Goldman, and Kornetsky 1967; Stein 1965.

presented a series of studies suggesting that central sympathomimetic systems produced "narrowed attention" (Callaway
and Dembo 1958; Callaway and Thompson 1953). I have
suggested that the so-called paradoxical effects of amphetamines in man (they act as stimulants in adults but can quiet
hyperactive children) are not truly paradoxical (1970). If
amphetamines act by increasing directed attention, task-
oriented attention, or secondary process at the expense of
primary process, this will appear as stimulation—increased
ability to concentrate, increased motivated learning, and so
on—in an adult already involved in secondary-process activities such as studying; but it will help to quiet a child whose
overactivity is based on distraction by peripheral stimuli or
by primary-process intrusion. Along these lines, my observations indicate that the effects of moderate doses of amphetamines in adults seem to include directed attention and also
strengthening of the subject's usual defensive patterns.

Stein (1965, 1967) has presented evidence, derived princi-
pally from studies on self-stimulation in rats, that catecholamine-containing neurons in the medial forebrain bundle may
comprise a reward system. This system is shown to be
involved not only in positive-reinforcement learning but in
certain aspects of avoidance learning as well, so that motivation or reinforcement may be considered an attribute of this
system, as well as "reward." Possibly related to this in man
are euphoria and increased motivation: amphetamine effects
in man have been summarized as producing, in addition to
and more prominently than an actually increased achieve-
ment on certain tasks, an increase in "need to achieve"
(Evans and Smith 1964).

In summary, there may be several separate but closely
interrelated affects and behaviors subserved by brain catecholamines: a tendency to optimistic or euphoric mood and
to increased "energy" and motivation; motor coordination;
new learning or short-term memory—especially reward systems and motivated learning; vigilance, attention, task orien-
tation, and secondary process; perhaps strengthened defen-

sive patterns; and need to achieve. These roles will be discussed again in terms of implication for "chemistry of the mind" (chapter 14, but for now it is apparent that the catecholamines play some role in integrated adaptive functioning during waking.

Implications for Functions of Sleep: A Hypothesis

Let us return to the inverse relationship I have outlined previously between brain catecholamines and D-time—that there may be a feedback mechanism connecting catecholamines and D-sleep such that conditions characterized by low catecholamines produce increased D-time, and that D-time in some way restores catecholamine levels or restores the integrity of the catecholaminergic brain systems, which as we have seen, play important roles during wakefulness (Hartmann 1970). I suggest the hypothesis that the drugs and clinical situations reviewed here, which greatly deplete brain catecholamines, may be seen as an exaggeration or parody of what happens during a normal day. In other words, normal waking may "wear out" certain systems, especially in the cortex, which depend on the ascending catecholamine pathways; and D-sleep may play a part in "restoring" them.

Are there other sorts of evidence for this hypothesis? First, as reviewed in chapter 4, there are studies indicating that D-deprivation appears to produce defects in new learning, focused attention, and normal psychological defenses—exactly those functions attributed above to the catecholaminergic systems. However, studies on these effects of D-deprivation have been difficult to control and to replicate. Likewise, the use of amphetamines in combating sleep deprivation may be cited as evidence, although it is not certain whether amphetamines counteract specifically the effects of D-deprivation; we have not yet studied this precisely in the laboratory. In animals there is a striking finding (Cohen and Dement 1965), which we have replicated (Stern and Hartmann 1972), that amphetamine lethality is reduced after

D-deprivation in animals. This is impressive because D-deprivation is, as mentioned, a stressful procedure, and after most stresses amphetamine lethality is clearly increased. This finding, therefore, strongly suggests that in D-deprivation the catecholamine systems especially stimulated by amphetamine are somehow less active, that perhaps receptors in this system are less sensitive.

It is also of interest that the typical hyperkinetic child, who is thought to have some defects in brain catecholamine systems (Wender 1971) and who responds dramatically to dextroamphetamine therapy, also resembles clinically a sleep-deprived or very tired child; he shows continually what the normal child will show under unusual circumstances when he is extremely tired (see chapter 11).

In connection with the studies we have reviewed showing that stimulation of the reticular activating system can produce subsequent increased D-time, one could study something similar using amphetamines, since amphetamines in effect produce a stimulation of the cortex through the reticular activating system. Previous studies have shown that amphetamines produce a reduced D-time with subsequent rebound, but this has always involved giving amphetamines at night, so that the organism is actually deprived of D-time which then appears to be "recovered." The present argument would suggest that even if amphetamines were given in the morning or at some time such that D-time was not reduced, there would nonetheless be a subsequent increase in D-time. In fact Small, Hibi, and Feinberg (1971) have done studies in 3 adults receiving 5 to 20mg of dextroamphetamine every morning; they reported a significant increase in D-time in all 3 subjects, even though 2 of the 3 had no suppression of D-time during administration.

More direct evidence might be sought by actually looking at synthesis and metabolism of catecholamines during D and S. Since these periods are extremely short in laboratory animals that can be readily studied chemically, we and other groups have chosen to study the condition of D-deprivation and the recovery periods following it that are perhaps exaggerations of conditions involving low D-time and conditions involving high D-time.

Pujol, Mouret, Jouvet, and Glowinski (1968), as well as our laboratory (Schildkraut and Hartmann 1972), have found that turnover of administered tritiated norepinephrine is clearly high during both deprivation and recovery periods. Our results disagree somewhat with theirs on recovery in that in our study the animals in the "continued D-deprivation" condition had the highest turnover rate, whereas they found the highest rates in the "recovery from D-deprivation" group. We found increased levels of norepinephrine during the recovery period, suggesting that synthesis rates were exceeding utilization rates. Most parsimoniously, we consider the results to be chiefly an effect of stress with no definite changes that must be attributed to the D-deprivation. However, it is quite possible that the D-deprivation followed by recovery represents an exaggeration of the normal stress of a day followed by a normal night's sleep. During a normal day, and perhaps increasingly during a stressful day, catecholamine turnover increases; then during the night, and especially during D-sleep, synthesis continues at a high level or perhaps even increases while utilization drops, so that there is an excess of synthesis over utilization.

We have also looked directly at tyrosine hydroxylase activity during D-deprivation and recovery from D-deprivation, since this is the rate-limiting enzyme in catecholamine synthesis, and at least one way in which D-time could assist in restoring or in increasing catecholamine levels would be to increase the synthesis or activation of tyrosine hydroxylase. The results show changes in the direction suggested—some reduction in enzyme activity in D-deprived animals (compared to similarly stressed controls) and some increase in enzyme activity in animals allowed to recover from D-deprivation; however, the percentage changes were not large (Hartmann and Popper 1972).

Another prediction from the hypothesis would be that

D-deprived animals might show a deficit in some of the waking functions requiring the catecholaminergic neuronal systems and that such deficits could be reversed at least temporarily by increasing available catecholamines. Several recent studies do demonstrate this effect. Stern (1969*a, b*) has shown that certain passive and active avoidance tasks show deterioration after D-deprivation and that this can be reversed by treatment with imipramine or pargyline. We have recently shown a similar reversal of D-deprivation effects with l-DOPA, the direct precursor of dopamine and norepinephrine (Hartmann and Stern 1972). We found that 4 days of D-deprivation produced a significant deficit in active avoidance conditioning. For unknown reasons, perhaps peripheral effects, l-DOPA alone also produced a considerable deficit in functioning on these tasks. However l-DOPA given after 4 days of D-deprivation returned learning function almost to normal levels (see table 8).[17]

It is of interest that in our studies of both AMPT and 6-hydroxydopamine the increases in D-time occurred at the expense of waking time, whiile S-sleep was unchanged. This increases the likelihood that, insofar as sleep has some functional role with regard to catecholamine systems, this may represent something like a balance between waking time and D-time, while S is perhaps not related in any way to the catecholamines.

This brings up the many ways in which D-sleep and waking have clear neurological similarities, whereas S is different. S is characterized by slow waves in the cortex and an inactive pattern in many forebrain areas, while both waking and D are characterized by desynchronized and in some ways activated patterns throughout, though there are of course differences between them. In a recent study Noda and Adey (1970) show that during S there is a good correlation between the firing

17. On a more general level D-deprivation produces a lowered convulsion threshold (Ferguson and Dement 1967), an effect very similar to that produced by reserpine and opposite to the effect produced by drugs which raise amine levels (Hartmann, Marcus, and Leinoff 1968).

Table 8. Active Avoidance Acquisition in the Rat
Number of Trials to Five Consecutive Avoidances ($\overline{X} \pm$ SEM)

Deprivation or Stress Condition		Drug Condition			
	No Drug	l-DOPA 200 mg/kg oral	AMPT 75 mg/kg oral	AMPT 75 mg/kg + l-DOPA 50–100 mg/kg	AMPT 75 mg/kg + l-DOPA 200 mg/kg
Normal	9.8 ± 1.6 (N = 19)	18.3 ± 1.8 (N = 11)	20.7 ± 1.7 (N = 12)	15.4 ± 2.8 (N = 8)	16.9 ± 1.5 (N = 17)
D-Deprivation 4 days	14.3 ± 1.8 (N = 15)	11.0 ± 1.4 (N = 10)	17.9 ± 2.9 (N = 7)	—	—
Water Stress 4 days	9.0 ± 1.4 (N = 11)	—	—	—	—

of the members of a neuronal pair, in single unit recordings recorded two at a time, whereas there is poor correlation between the two neurons in waking and in D. This appears consistent with the view we are developing that waking is, obviously, an active state characterized by excitation, learning, and memory formation, and that in D-sleep there is a sort of *reworking* or *rearousal* of the same areas, pathways, and mechanisms.

If indeed, as I have suggested, the functioning of catecholaminergic systems is improved or restored during sleep and during D-sleep especially, precisely how could this be accomplished? There are several possibilities, and data is not yet available to decide among them. (1) The synthesis of catecholamines in relevant neurons may actually be increased. Since tyrosine hydroxylase is considered the rate-limiting step, this enzyme could be involved, particularly since its activity has been shown to be responsive to stress and to drugs such as reserpine. We have shown suggestive but not conclusive evidence of this in D-deprived animals. (2) There are various mechanisms by which catecholamines at brain synapses could be rendered more active: by preventing reuptake into cells, by stimulation of release, or by preventing enzymatic catabolism of the amines. This is the way some antidepressant medication and other drugs are thought to function, and we have discussed similarities between these and what happens during D; however, I do not consider it very likely that the complex neurological events occurring during D are involved with such potentially rapid mechanisms for increasing synaptic availability of catecholamines. (3) There is a possibility that the receptors for catecholamines somehow become less sensitive during the day and are restored during D or that the presynaptic axonal endings, with their storage vesicles, or the tubules used in channeling catecholamines to the endings, are somehow restored. These mechanisms, which could be called structural restoration, all would involve synthesis and laying down of new structural as well as perhaps enzymatic protein. This third possibility appears to me to be the most likely guess as to the mechanisms involved in the postulated restoration.

It is possible that electron microscope studies could directly differentiate between the above possibilities, but I have been assured by experts that it will be some years before studies are precise enough for such investigations involving small neurons in the densely populated cerebral cortex and catecholamine-containing axonal endings, which are very difficult to detect individually.

In the preceding chapters we have seen that psychologically we might visualize D-time as having a role in restoring the mind or brain after intense new learning or difficult stressful or emotional experiences; on the physiological level the same result may occur after intense stimulation of the reticular activating system; and on the chemical level, after situations which produce decreases in functional brain catecholamines. Is it possible that these various levels are all related or in fact refer to the same conditions? I would suggest that an emotionally and intellectually tiring day is a day which has involved unusual bombardment of the cortex and higher nervous centers by the reticular activating system, and is a day in which the catecholamine synapses, probably at the cortex, become especially worn out or ineffective. Sleep and specifically D-sleep could then be seen as providing recuperation for these catecholamine-dependent neuron systems involved in learning, memory, attention, and emotional equilibrium during waking.

In surveying the pharmacological data, I have spoken about *catecholamines,* since most of the studies cannot differentiate between norepinephrine and dopamine. However, in terms of a hypothesis I can be more specific and suggest that the "catecholamine systems" I am speaking of consist of the ascending norepinephrine bundles (especially the "dorsal bundle") and their cortical terminations.

These studies also suggest that synchronized sleep, which is increased after physical exercise, possibly after pain and physical injury, and after certain hypermetabolic conditions in which body tissues are "burned up," may reasonably have an anabolic restorative function, possibly needed by the entire body, not only the brain.

11 The Psychology of Tiredness

We have already discussed sleep deprivation, and this has taught us something about the functions of sleep; but sleep deprivation is an artificial, stressful condition, occurring in a complex social-experimental setting. In many human sleep-deprivation situations the subject has a desire to perform well; especially if he is in a group, there is an ésprit de corps that can produce good performance in spite of sleep deprivation. This is particularly true in laboratory sleep-deprivation experiments, where the subject is challenged, mobilizes his defenses, and has a "set" to perform well. When sleep deprivation is used in a different setting, for instance as part of a "marathon" group dynamics session, the set is rather to regress and to become more "open"; here very different results are found. All behavioral sleep-deprivation results are thus heavily influenced by the setting and expectations.

I will now turn to a related situation which is closer to our everyday experience—simple tiredness. By tiredness I do not mean the fatigue after exercise, from which one recovers merely by lying down without sleeping, but the tiredness at the end of a day, apparently reversible only by sleep. One approach to the functions of sleep is to examine carefully the state of tiredness and to determine what characteristics or structures of the mind appear to wear out during the day and to need restoration by sleep. A study of what happens during a day as one becomes increasingly tired suffers from none of the above problems connected with experimental sleep deprivation; on the other hand, tiredness might be expected to produce less marked or obvious changes than prolonged sleep deprivation.

It is surprising how little has been written that can be useful to us here. Although a number of books and articles exist apparently dealing with tiredness or fatigue,[1] they

1. Bartley 1965; Dodge 1917; Morris 1967; Seham and Seham 1926.

usually consider the muscular aspects and say almost nothing about the psychology of tiredness. Nonetheless, it is perfectly obvious both from our own subjective experience and from observation of other persons, especially children, that considerable changes in psychological functioning are produced by tiredness, and these are what we shall examine here.

This chapter necessarily will be clinical and somewhat impressionistic, and findings will be conceptualized in psychiatric and psychoanalytic terms.[2] What I will discuss here is based on experience with patients in psychotherapy and psychoanalysis, several hundred interviews with normal and abnormal sleepers in various sleep studies, observation of children, and introspection. The chief problem lies in attempting to extricate constant themes from the changing, variegated clinical material, for the effects of tiredness clearly depend to a great extent on the background mental characteristics of the person, as well as on his social and physical environment.

Nonetheless, it appears to me that two patterns or "syndromes" of tiredness can be identified (see table 9). They are seldom present in pure form, and not everyone reports both types, but a large number of individuals, when they stop to think about it, can pick out these two very different characteristic sorts of tiredness in themselves. One is the tiredness that comes after a day of purely physical activity, such as a day of skiing or physical work. This could be called physical tiredness or simple tiredness and is associated usually with a relaxed feeling in the musculature, including the facial and head muscles, and very seldom with any tightness or headaches. It is usually described affectively as either pleasant or neutral and is not associated with any characteristic psychic changes: people find it difficult to say that their mental functioning was altered in this kind of tiredness. In children

2. If the reader unfamiliar with psychoanalytic terms will bear with me through a few phrases such as "economic point of view" or "structural point of view" which cannot be defined in a brief space, I believe he will nonetheless find my conclusions easy to understand.

Table 9. Two Kinds of Tiredness Requiring Sleep

	Tiredness 1	*Tiredness 2*
Rough Designation	"Physical"	"Mental"
Typically Follows	A day of physical activity, sport, or mixed physical-intellectual activity without worry or anxiety	A day of emotional stress or a day of hard, not entirely pleasant, intellectual work or intellectual plus emotional work
Muscles	Usually relaxed	Often tense
Physical Symptoms	None	Sometimes headache, eye strain, or cramped or tense feelings in various muscles
Affective Tone	Neutral or pleasant	Neutral or, often, unpleasant
Sleep Onset	Rapid, easy	Sometimes slow, difficult
Mental Changes (Adult)	No definite changes	Discomfort, irritability, anger, lack of energy, inability to concentrate, loss of social adaptiveness, loss of ability for careful patterning or long term planning
Mental Changes (Children)	No definite changes	Regression, loss of superego, emergence of naked anger or hostility, temper tantrums, "too tired to get to sleep"
Metapsychological Formulation	No change	Wearing out of the most recently developed or most subtle ego mechanisms, wearing out of secondary process, emergence of drive and impulses, especially anger
Hypothesized Relationship to Sleep	Represents a "need" for SWS	Represents a "need" for D

my impression is that this physical tiredness is associated with relaxation and with rapid sleep onset without fuss or bother.

The second kind of tiredness, which we might call mental tiredness, is reported more frequently after a long day of intellectual or emotional and intellectual work. This tiredness, with which most of us are all too familiar, is often accompanied by tension or tightness of the muscles, especially muscles of the face and head; and it is usually described with a negative tone—it is unpleasant or at best neutral. It sometimes has the paradoxical effect of making it hard to fall asleep.[3] Associated with this sort of tiredness is an obvious lack of energy or unwillingness to try anything new; irritability and anger are also prominent. One feels uncomfortable and on edge in social interactions and wants to be left alone in an undemanding situation. One tends to read easy material and to lapse into wish-fulfilling daydreams.

The following are some of the words and phrases people have used in describing themselves, their friends, or their children at times when I believe they are discussing this second kind of tiredness: "cranky, impatient, selfish, dissatisfied, feel cuddly, want support, think loosely, sensuous, crying, stubborn, loss of energy, quick to anger, depressed, unaccepting, less sense of power, less self-confidence, more babyish, hate to be disturbed, don't want to think, can't think in a concentrated fashion, want to read easy material, I want what I want when I want it, want to be patted, less superego, less idealistic, more grabby, more selfish, very aggressive, hard to control, perseverates, repeats the same phrases or actions, temper tantrums, refuses to get to sleep although very tired, unwilling to act, less feeling of freedom, poor social functioning, poor adaptation, more denial of painful reality, distractible, hard to keep attention centered, hard to stick to one subject for long, unable to change mind, a little paranoid, less need to achieve, less control, less integration."

3. MacCurdy, many years ago (1920), described something like this as one variety of insomnia.

The above are very general effects of this sort of tiredness. The exact effects obviously vary with the individual's personality structure. In some persons with a tendency toward depression, increasing depression is characteristic of tiredness, and they may even go to sleep to avoid depression. For others (especially certain patients with sleep-onset insomnia) the great problem in becoming tired is the feeling of losing control, losing one's normal ways of dealing with sexual and especially aggressive impulses.

This second sort of tiredness clearly involves alterations in psychic functions, a tiring of the psychic apparatus; but I believe that not every aspect of mental functioning tires equally. In cognitive fields this tiredness expresses itself as a difficulty in concentration, especially in sustained attentive thinking, and also as a defect in exclusion of extraneous or unwanted stimuli.

In children there are clear evidences of ego regression. As the day wears on to evening there is a striking inability to control impulses and wishes. The child becomes more of a baby as he becomes tired. For instance, a four-year-old boy who has learned perfectly that hitting his younger sister when he is angry at her is not tolerable and has learned to displace and to sublimate his impulse, nonetheless reverts to simply hitting her when he is extremely tired. Also, when small children are very tired, there are frequent instances of verbal perseveration—using the same phrases to make the same demands over and over again. This is perhaps a regression to one of the earliest psychic tendencies—the repetition compulsion. The general impression both in children and adults is that more subtle and more recently developed ego mechanisms are the ones which tire most easily.

From the economic point of view mental tiredness means that less psychic energy is available for higher-level activities, such as directed conscious attention; and there is a greater mobility of cathexes. Secondary-process functioning tires especially, sometimes allowing primary process to emerge. In the conflict-free sphere lowered energy shows up as poor

attention and decreased activity-directed energy. In con-
flictual spheres lowered energy for countercathexes produces
regression, impulsivity, and less subtle and adaptive handling
of drives, especially aggressive drive.

From the structural point of view there is not much
evidence that the id becomes tired. It appears likely that the
drives maintain their strength but that the mechanisms in the
ego which normally deal with these drives tire and become
less effective. It seems to me that the more subtle and, in
children, the more recently developed ego mechanisms tire
the most. The ego ideal and the superego are among the
structures which tire easily, especially in children where they
are only recently or incompletely formed.

From the dynamic point of view there is a weakening in the
ego defense mechanisms for dealing with drives and with
reality, and a regression to earlier "easier" mechanisms. The
forms this regression takes vary with the characteristics of the
individual. (I do not believe that there is always a clear-cut
libidinal regression, although this may also occur with a
choice of earlier modes, for instance oral modes, of gratifica-
tion.)[4] One could also conceptualize what deteriorates during
tiredness as the careful balance of the ego in which the drives
guarantee the ego's autonomy from outside reality and reality
guarantees the ego's autonomy from the drives (Rapaport
1950). In the normal individual the ego maintains a smooth
balance, hopefully not requiring too much energy, between
the demands of the external world and the demands of its
own drives. When very tired, a small child often, and the
adult sometimes, will be taken over by his more primitive
wishes and desires: I want this, I want that, I want what I
want, and so on. The adult's aggression often takes over
during extreme tiredness and overrides generally well-learned
social amenities. On the other hand, in the adult, in whom the

4. The previously mentioned paradoxical difficulty in falling asleep though
very tired arises when the increasing regression, primary process, and so on
are sensed as a dangerous loss of control.

demands of reality are sometimes extremely strong, the balance often tips the other way in extreme tiredness, so that rather than feeling overwhelmed by one's drives, one feels entirely overwhelmed by the outside world, by the amount of work needed to be done, by external demands, and so on. It is the balance which appears to be lacking.

In adaptive terms the psyche can be seen as regressing during tiredness, as gradually relinquishing its attempts to deal with the more demanding aspects of reality (both cognitive and affective) and slowly adapting to a diminishing, simpler, less demanding reality.

In a "guidance system" [5] framework tiredness, especially the second kind of tiredness, seems to involve difficulty in maintaining subtle feedback-controlled mechanisms. The body can be seen as an extremely delicate set of balances and homeostatic adjustments, each delicately tuned and each generally in a state of stable equilibrium; this is especially true of the central nervous system. Tiredness affects these balanced mechanisms so that there is a less delicate balance or tuning. In extreme tiredness there is less of the usual delicate "buffering": a small external input can produce a large perturbation which is not immediately and smoothly damped out as it would normally be. I relate this sort of buffering to the activity of ascending catecholamine systems, perhaps acting at the cortical level (see chapter 14); tiredness then represents inadequate function of these systems.

Although nothing can be proved conclusively from the evidence presented here, the implications for function are clear. We have delineated psychologically two kinds of tiredness which, in turn, suggests two restorative functions— one relatively simple and physical, the other involving restoration of subtle adaptive ego functions, which can also be seen as feedback guidance processes. From what has gone

5. The term *guidance system* implies an analogy between the mental apparatus which guides the individual through environmental (including social) time and space and the system which guides a space vehicle through physical space. This will be discussed again later.

before the reader will not be surprised at my suggestion that the first, relatively simple, "physical tiredness" represents a need for slow wave sleep (stages 3–4), while the second, more complex, "mental tiredness" represents a need for D-sleep. In the normal course of events a night's sleep fills both of these needs.

12 The Dream and the Functions of Sleep

In formulating, from many different points of view, certain psychological and physiological functions for the D-state, I have so far neglected one of its most striking manifestations, the one which in fact historically led to such widespread interest in this phase of sleep—the experience of dreaming. I shall make no attempt to review or even summarize our total knowledge about the dream, or even the considerable knowledge that has derived in the last few years from laboratory sleep studies. I shall restrict myself here to the question of whether an examination of the manifest dream can give us further hints as to sleep functions. Has the dream itself anything to teach us about the functions of sleep?

One extreme hypothesis would be that the experience of dreaming may itself be the major function of sleep and that the role of sleep may be merely to allow a state such that dreams may emerge. Although Freud never made such a statement, some have interpreted Freud in this light. French and Fromm (1964), Jones (1962), and others have suggested an adaptive or ego-growth–promoting function for dreams and have implied that sleep may exist chiefly to allow dreams to occur.

My own impression is, first, that the recall of dream content cannot be of importance in the functions of sleep— that the functional roles of sleep and dreaming sleep are fulfilled whether or not any dreams are actually recalled. So many incidental factors—spontaneous awakenings, restless sleep, conscious interest in dreams, even laboratory awakenings—can greatly alter the amount of dream recall but have little effect on the basic biology of sleep; and such alterations do not appear to have striking psychological effects. Furthermore, it is obvious that many persons never recall dreams at all and that others only recall dreams at certain times of their lives, when they happen to be waking frequently during the night, for instance, or happen to be interested in dreams. It seems probable that whatever adaptive function sleep may have cannot be restricted by such haphazard considerations. Thus I suspect that dreaming sleep has a function quite independent of what one recalls about one's dreams.[1]

The experienced dream, even if it is not the raison d'être of sleep, is of interest to us here in its role as a *concomitant* or *indicator* of important events taking place in the brain (see also chapter 14). In other words, I think that sleep, including D-sleep, has certain functions outlined previously and that the experienced manifest dream, when present, is a sort of window into these processes; dreaming consciousness "looks in" briefly at various bits of the mental process of connections being formed, as waking consciousness "looks in" on small portions of the great variety of processes that may be going on at any one time during waking. I believe that the psychological experience of dreaming, like any psychic experience (PSI-state), cannot be studied scientifically in its own right, but rather as an *indicator* of what may be going on—whether what is going on is conceptualized psychologically (say in psychoanalytic metapsychology) or physiologically.[2] Such an indicator can be an important tool, and I think it quite possible that the structure of the dream as we know it can lead to some useful insights as to the functions of sleep and that some striking aspects of dreaming phenomenology can be related, as indicators, to physiological events suggested previously.

Condensation and Central Nodal Images

As one example, let us consider the striking aspect of dream structure called *condensation,* in which one manifest

1. This does not of course mean that dream recall, the exchange of information about dreams, analysis of dreams, and so on cannot in themselves play additional functional roles during waking, but this is completely separate from the functions of sleep.

2. I have discussed this view in detail (Hartmann 1966c; see also chapter 14). It is basically the same view proposed by Hughlings Jackson (1932) among others, that psychic events are related as concomitants to the simultaneous physiological events.

dream element appears as a merging of two or more images or thoughts and derives from two or more mental pathways (latent dream thoughts) present at the same time. Such an element could indicate new connections of some kind being formed or tested between previously unconnected material. In other words, a manifest dream element analyzable as a condensation of two latent thoughts or themes is an indicator that two pathways are being connected or brought together. It is reasonable that a new piece of input from waking life is often connected with an old brain pathway to which it is in some way related. (Or, in psychoanalytic terms, a manifest dream element derives from a day residue plus an old wish or fear it has "aroused.") More generally, primary process in dreaming—primitive connections, large discharges of energy, opposites occurring together—can all be seen as characteristics of a "reconnecting" process in which daytime residues are reconnected to large, old, and thus "primitive" pathways or brain storage systems.

Similarly, let us consider the single very vivid image that sometimes stands out in a dream. Freud speaks of an overdetermination of each element in the dream and especially of the more vivid elements—which may represent condensation of three or more latent thoughts. I would suggest that such an element may indicate a nodal point representing interconnections between multiple brain pathways which somehow achieve enough prominence to be noticed by dreaming consciousness.

Thus the overall hypothesis I am proposing is that during D-sleep new connections are formed, especially in cortical areas served by ascending catecholamine pathways, and that specifically new connections are formed between daytime memories that have somehow been left unconnected and old pathways. This is entirely compatible with Freud's formulation that dreams are made up of day residue material and old wishes. However, I would add that it need not necessarily be *wishes,* although certainly old wishes and fears may be among the primary and most primitive channels for forming connections,[3] and during dreams daytime material is connected to these old systems or channels.

The Dream as a Story

Some well-known aspects of the structure of the manifest dream have been used above to indicate underlying processes; perhaps this can be done with other less-known characteristics of the dream as well. A very prominent but frequently neglected aspect of dreaming is that the dream usually unrolls as a kind of story sequence or sometimes as a number of different stories. The stories subjectively take a certain amount of time, and dreams have in fact been shown objectively to take time—approximately as much time as the events would take in waking life (Dement and Wolpert 1958). Dreams do *not* consist of constant kaleidoscopic shifts among disconnected elements nor do they take any number of forms which waking thought sometimes takes, i.e., questions and answers, philosophical conceptual discussions, and so on. A dream often consists of the introduction of an unusual or bizarre element or situation, followed by relatively normal story development for a period of seconds or minutes, until a sudden switch of scene or introduction of a new vivid element occurs. It is chiefly the specific bizarre or unusual events which stand out and are interpreted and which appear to be produced by condensation, displacement, and so on. We have considered these vivid elements above; let us now concentrate on the less-noticed story-unfolding aspect of dreams, again as a possible indicator of underlying processes.

The story-sequence quality of the dream certainly suggests that some storage and retrieval processes may occur in short story sequences arrayed in approximately proper temporal arrangement. This sort of storage is suggested also by the

3. Rapaport (1951) has referred to the child's first memory system as "drive-organization of memory."

work of Penfield and Jasper (1954), who have found exactly this temporal property for memories they have been able to elicit by cortical stimulation during brain surgery in conscious waking patients. They found that a single short stimulation in the temporal cortex produces a whole story from memory, which unfolds to the patient in proper temporal sequence over a space of seconds or minutes. Others have reported that stimulation produces a shift of sequence or a shift to more primary process without determining a specific memory sequence (Mahl, Rothenberg, Delgado, and Hamlin 1961).

The breaks in sequence or shifts in thought from one series of images to another have recently been shown to be associated with electrically measurable phasic eye-muscle events in man,[4] which are apparently related to the PGO spikes in the cat (Watson 1972). Perhaps these impulses, reaching the cortex, somehow jar the systems involved and switch consciousness to another series of connections in the process of being laid down. This switch or rapid leap to distant paths is certainly an aspect of primary process. In terms of brain function we could see PGO spikes, the phasic events of the D-periods, as instructions to cement or to test a new connection being formed; this new nodal point, or one of the new ones thus activated, would then suddenly appear in consciousness. Perhaps these sporadic brain discharges, arriving at the cortex from the brain stem, act somewhat like Penfield's or Mahl's occasional successes with external stimulation and produce a shift of focus, followed by a train of memory. If so, then the characteristic dream sequence—the sudden appearance of a prominent element followed by a relatively straightforward story in temporal sequence—would "indicate," at the cortical level, an impulse arriving, forming or cementing a node or connection, followed by more ordinary sequential activation of memory sequences.[5]

4. These are known as phasic integrated potentials (PIPs).
5. Or rather a memorylike sequence to incorporate the unusual or bizarre element. The cementing or connection produces condensation and the

What Is Not in the Dream

I have tried another related approach to the question of whether the dream can indicate something that is going on functionally in the brain. I have suggested previously that what occurs during sleep, especially during D-sleep, is the formation and testing of new connections as part of a process of repair and restoration of certain catecholamine-dependent brain systems that are necessary during waking. If this is true, then one might expect that these particular systems are not functioning normally during dreaming and that in some sense they may be "shunted out" for repairs. It might be interesting again to use the dream as an indicator, but now to ask what psychological functions or capacities are *missing* in the dream, to see whether these may correspond in some way to the waking systems I am suggesting are being repaired. Therefore, I have tried, with help from other psychiatrists and psychologists, to formulate exactly what does *not* occur in dreams—what cognitive or emotional processes occur during waking and not during dreaming.

First of all, in terms of pure sensory experience, there is nothing obvious which does not occur in dreams although, clearly, dreaming consciousness is shifted in the direction of more visual experience.

Emotions occur in dreaming as well as in waking, but it appears that the simpler and more primitive emotions predominate in dreams, while the softer or subtler, more adult emotions seem to be lost. Also, the feeling of being tired or of being energetic and alert are seldom experienced as such in dreams, though they are very common in waking life. As I have emphasized elsewhere, the feeling of free will, so prominent in waking life, seems to be absent or almost totally

---

striking dream element; the memorylike device then takes over and provides an unremarkable sort of continuation. The process seems to accept the unusual event or situation and then continues in terms of what is likely to happen on the basis of available memories.

absent in dreams (Hartmann 1966c). Also usually missing in dreams are emotions which depend on feedback from the environment—for instance, the feeling of anger which changes gradually to sympathy depending on a turn that a conversation may be taking. However, very sudden dramatic shifts do occur; one seldom maintains the same steady emotion throughout a dream. In other words, some sort of continuous feeling of the self is not present in dreams. One does not feel oneself as an entity existing through time, having free will, and interacting emotionally with the environment.

In terms of cognitive processes there is certainly less hard, concentrated, logical thinking in dreams than in waking, but thinking does occur. However, attention processes are obviously altered in some way. One thing that is lacking in dreams is prolonged concentrated attention on a task; one is unable to concentrate on one item and avoid distraction by others. Also, the ability to shift attention rapidly and to be able to pay attention simultaneously or in rapid sequence to a number of different persons or items in one's environment appears not to be present in dreams. This may merely be stating that one has less control over attention and over other capacities.

Furthermore, a series of processes involved in relating oneself to one's environment over time are lacking in the dream. Thus the usual feedback processing, the testing of "patterns" in the environment, and the whole dynamic feedback "guidance system" enabling one to interact with and test one's surroundings are missing. In fact, time and space seem less well organized in the dream. The edges of the visual dream space are imprecise, and one is half unaware of time. Kant called time and space the pure forms of our perception ("sensual intuition"); these means of patterning are, again, missing or distorted in dreams.

Also, a very obvious aspect of dreams, often overlooked because it is so obvious, is the degree of acceptance of bizarre or unusual events, in other words, the lack of surprise at anything that may happen. Here again there is an entire faculty which is shut off during the dream, a higher ego function having to do with precise reality testing or judgment.

My suggestion, obviously speculative at this point, is that those functions enumerated above, which occur in waking but *not* in dreaming, are functions of the cortex under the influence of the catecholaminergic neuronal systems; these I see as being repaired during sleep and perhaps "shunted out" for purposes of repair and reworking; thus the dream can show us the functioning of the brain when the catecholamine influence is removed. Evidence that the catecholamines may be involved in many of these mental activities (energy, free will, sense of self, focused attention, patterning) has been reviewed elsewhere (Hartmann 1970; see also chapter 10).[6] Additionally, the lack of "continuing sense of self" is exactly the defect described by Robinson and Freeman (1954) as the most prominent overall characteristic of postlobotomy patients, who presumably have a more permanent disconnection of some of the cortical systems we are considering. In other words, the more primitive, primary-process–dominated activity, *not* involving the aspects above, is perhaps the way the systems function when the catecholamine influences are disconnected or not being used. This state is found in dreaming, and of course can be partly experienced under certain waking conditions, such as acute psychosis and drug-induced states. Also, as we have seen, tiredness and sleep-deprivation can lead to somewhat dreamlike thought and consciousness even when awake; in other words, these conditions can result in poor functioning of the same systems that I see as entirely missing in the dream.

Differences among Dreams

Can we learn anything about the functions of sleep by observing changes in dreams within a person or differences in

6. The amphetamines, which act by releasing catecholamines, are, in other words, intensifiers of catecholamine activity and produce a temporary *increase* or intensification in these same functions which are absent in dreams.

dreams between persons? Could the alterations in dreams across a night be used as indicators of any underlying process? Perhaps the increase in emotionality and the increased references to a subject's distant past in later dreams of the night (Foulkes 1966; Verdone 1965) are compatible with the idea of brain connections being formed at deeper and deeper levels as the night progresses.

Can differences in dream experience between persons or within persons at different times be used as indicators of important underlying differences? Here it might be worth looking again at the long, short, and variable sleepers. The long sleepers reported more dreams at home, had longer dream reports in the laboratory, and were obviously more involved in their dreams; also, the long sleepers, on an objective scale, had more primary process in their dreams than did the short sleepers. This may be connected to the fact that the long sleepers appeared to require far more D-time; they seemed to have considerable worries and engaged in constant reprogramming, suggesting that the whole process of restoration and reconnections during D is psychologically more important to them than to the short sleepers.

Since many factors influence the amount of dream recall, it is difficult to be certain, but I now believe that there is usually more dream recall, and of a more vivid, dreamlike nature, at the times I have characterized as requiring more sleep or more D-time—routinely in the long sleepers as opposed to normal or short sleepers; at times of stress, mild depression, and change in variable sleepers; during the premenstrual period in women with premenstrual tension, and so on (see chapters 5, 6, and 7).

The increased amount of dreaming, increased primary process, dreamlike quality, and so on all indicate that more of what we have suggested as the work of sleep and especially of D-sleep is being performed. Since we are assuming that the dream gives an indication as to what is being connected, it looks as though in these situations deeper, more far-reaching, or more profound connections are being made; and, reasonably, these do appear to occur at times when deep or difficult material has been stirred up during the day.[7]

Implications for Functions of Sleep

In this chapter we have seen that the structure of the manifest dream itself can be employed as an indicator which can lead us to some aspects of underlying processes important in the functions of sleep. I suggest that aspects of the structure of the manifest dream are at least consistent with the same processes and functions that we have hypothesized starting from very different sorts of data—the possible repair of certain waking systems involving focused attention, free will, energy, secondary process, and so on, and the formation of connections in memory systems, especially connections between recently acquired material that has remained unassimilated and older memory pathways. Further, I have speculated that a careful study of waking functions absent in dreaming may tell us something about what waking functions may be "resting" or being "repaired" during sleep. It appears that these waking functions involve focused attention, finding and imposing patterns, and careful feedback modulated self-guidance. Certainly this examination of the dream does not provide any proof of my hypotheses on the functions of

7. The material from the day that is left over and needs to be incorporated during D-periods is generally material that is meaningful in terms of the person's own life and psychodynamics, and those are the elements which make for especially vivid, emotional dreams. Thus, for instance, laboratory dreams obtained under routine conditions usually turn out to be fairly dull and unemotional (Snyder 1967). Even dreams obtained after the showing of anxiety-provoking films were still relatively routine, even though they did at times incorporate elements of the film (Witkin and Lewis 1967). On the other hand, extremely vivid, emotional, personal laboratory dreams were obtained by Breger, Hunter, and Lane (1971) in a situation where the dreamer was a member of a therapy group and had been placed on the "hot seat" and made the subject of discussion the evening just before collection of laboratory dreams. In these situations there was clearly a great deal of personal, emotional material stirred up during the session which needed to be handled by the dreamer in some way.

sleep. I have merely suggested some new ways of looking at dream content and, using these, have found evidence at least compatible with the previously developed views on function.

III. SUMMARY AND IMPLICATIONS

13   The Functions of Sleep: Summary

I have now reviewed many facts about sleep and suggested hints about functions of sleep derived from a number of data bases and channels of exploration. From all these points of departure, we have arrived at views of the functions of sleep which are at least coherent and which can be seen as referring to the same overall theory of function. This theory is, I believe, compatible with the major classes of facts about sleep that are known at present and has also been fruitful to me and my collaborators in suggesting many new areas of exploration. This to my mind makes it plausible and useful, which does not however mean that it is true or necessarily the only explanation for the facts, and it certainly does not imply that, if true, it is a complete explanation of the functions of sleep.

I shall review here the findings relevant to function from the fields already examined and the major tenets of the theory of the functions of sleep I am proposing. I shall then attempt to show that this theory accounts for most aspects of the phenomenology of sleep reviewed earlier.

In summarizing the material reviewed, there has been no reason to question that sleep basically has a restitutive or restorative function, in accordance with our commonsense notions. Sleep is required by all persons and by all mammals, and apparently there are separable requirements for the two major states of sleep (see figure 15).

Functions of S-Sleep

Let me consider first what we have discovered about possible functions of S-sleep. From what has gone before it is likely that slow-wave sleep (SWS), the deeper and probably most intensive part of S-sleep, has a physically restorative function, which is more necessary after exercise or when

145

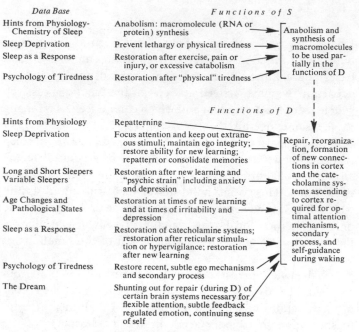

Figure 15. The functions of sleep.

catabolism has been increased. One could consider SWS an anabolic phase of sleep. On the basis of the tentative evidence described, I would suggest that SWS could be a phase when macromolecules—proteins and/or RNA—are synthesized, especially in the central nervous system. These macromolecules are then used partly in the functions of D. Although the increased requirements for SWS may be produced by states of general body tiredness or increased catabolism, the increased synthetic processes probably occur especially in the brain. It is brain electrophysiology that dramatically differentiates SWS from relaxed wakefulness, and I also believe SWS plays an additional preparatory role for the functions of D in the brain.

Functions of D-Sleep

Functions of D have been discussed in more detail; these appear clearly to involve the central nervous system and to be more complex than the functions of S. From the studies of sleep deprivation and the studies of tiredness we have concluded that sleep, and probably D-sleep specifically, may have a restorative function with respect to systems of focused attention (especially the ability to focus on one item while ignoring others); systems involving the ability to maintain an optimistic mood, energy, and self-confidence; and systems involving processes of emotional adaptation to the physical and social environment.

From the studies of long, short, and variable sleepers we have concluded that sleep, especially D-sleep, is needed in larger quantities after days of stress, worry, or intense new learning, especially if the learning is in itself somewhat stressful. D-sleep thus may have a role in consolidating learning or memory, but there is a strong hint that stress is important and that more D is needed when there have been emotionally involving changes during the day. In other words, those who require more sleep are not so much persons who have learned a lot of new facts during the day, but rather persons who have disrupted their usual ways of doing things, who have, often stressfully, reprogrammed themselves during their waking hours. Thus sleep and D-sleep may have a role in consolidating or reconnecting these important alterations made during the day. Thinking of psychodynamic concepts in somewhat too literal a sense, one can almost see psychic structures, when they are tried out in new ways (at times of stress), rubbing against each other and producing friction and then requiring increased restoration by sleep; while these same mechanisms, when they are functioning smoothly, can handle a great deal of input without requiring much sleep for restoration.

Investigations as to what systems were not observable during dreaming and thus might be in the process of repair led to some of the same systems (focused attention, energy, etc.) and, more especially, the overall sense of guidance of the self—feedback-interactive self-guidance—associated with a continuing sense of self over time. This concept might unify some of the psychological mechanisms listed above, since certainly self-guidance over time requires focused attention, ability to include and exclude stimuli, ability to see patterns in the environment, ability for social interaction, as well as enough positive mood and self-confidence to keep these processes going. Our examination of the psychology of tiredness has enabled me to suggest that to a large extent the same processes that wear out during tiredness are the ones which are entirely absent during dreaming. These processes, which I suggest are restored during D-sleep, are the ones whose physiology and chemistry we can then try to specify.

On a physiological level it appears that an animal with a cortex has more sleep than an animal without a cortex and that sleep and especially D-time can be increased by several hours of intensive stimulation of the reticular activating system, perhaps similar to intensive new learning in animals or in man. Thus the systems that may tire and require more sleep and more D-time for restoration quite likely involve the cerebral cortex, certainly including the frontal lobes, as well as perhaps ascending pathways from the midbrain to the cortex. (I have suggested, specifically, the catecholamine-containing pathways ascending from the midbrain in several fluorometrically discernible bundles, corresponding to portions of the ascending medial forebrain bundle.)

From chemical and pharmacological studies I have presented evidence that low catecholamine levels increase D-time, while high catecholamine levels tend to reduce D-time; it is possible, then, that desynchronized sleep has a homeostatic feedback role in restoring brain catecholamines or catecholamine-containing systems. I consider the drug-induced low-catecholamine situation to be an inexact parody of what normally occurs during the day, and I would say that the function of D-sleep might be to restore adequate conditions in catecholaminergic systems and their cortical endings rather than to replete some hypothetical amine pool in the brain. These catecholamine-containing systems involve especially the medial forebrain bundle and its extensions forward to the cortex. It is still unclear whether it is the catecholaminergic synapses that are important; it is quite possible that release of catecholamines in cortical regions and the general diffusion of the amines there may have a modulatory effect such as has been suggested by Kety (1970), aside from any direct synaptic effect.[1]

The restoration of these cortical systems and corticopetal systems could be accomplished in several ways, as mentioned in chapter 10. First, D-sleep could facilitate actual synthesis of the catecholamines, and we have investigated this in the study of tyrosine hydroxylase activity. This would fit with the time intervals of minutes or hours: the protein hypothetically synthesized during S could be further altered leading to specific enzymes such as tyrosine hydroxylase, or this enzyme could be activated, or placed in position, during D-sleep. However this particular mechanism does not seem especially consistent with the memory and reconnection function we have also postulated. Second, catecholaminergic systems could be restored by some simple synaptic mechanism such as altering membrane reuptake or catabolism of amines in the synaptic cleft. These, however, are often short-term mechanisms which would not particularly require hours of sleep; further, these effects are produced by antidepressant drugs which do not have the "restorative" properties of sleep. And again, such a mechanism does not explain the postulated memory reconnections. Third, receptor mechanisms or other aspects of the physical structure of the synapse might be changed in order to render it again more sensitive to catecholamines or more efficacious in its activity. This seems

1. Presumably there must be cortico-reticular systems which monitor the state of the cortex—its "alertness," amounts of norepinephrine release, and so on—and then relay this into the brain stem to enhance or suppress D-time.

to me to be the most attractive possibility because, in addition to making use of proteins or other macromolecules previously synthesized and requiring at least the length of time actually involved, the restructuring of synapses is definitely a mechanism by which cortical systems depending on catecholamines not only could be restored to previous sensitivity, but also could be altered by changing conductivity or formation of new connections; this of course could easily be related to the reconnecting and memory functions we have discussed. Although this third view is perhaps the most reasonable, it unfortunately does not lend itself to direct experimental verification at this point. Electron microscopy of small uniform cells, such as the cortical neurons, and their synaptic structure is still in a developmental stage; and there is no certain way of locating specifically the presynaptic endings of ascending catecholamine neurons in electron microscopy. Search by these means therefore is not yet indicated, although in a few years it may be entirely possible. I can think of no other direct way of looking at this suggested mechanism, though many indirect means have been discussed in the course of this book.

Thus on a chemical basis I have suggested that D-sleep could function in the restoration—perhaps by means of synaptic rebuilding, using macromolecules previously synthesized—of the catecholamine-dependent systems which play a role in psychological mechanisms including attention, secondary process, and guidance during waking (figure 15). It is obvious that I am engaged in the necessary but somewhat dangerous occupation of erecting several hypotheses depending on each other; aside from hypotheses about the functions of sleep, I am proposing certain functions for the catecholamines in the brain, which will be discussed further in chapter 14.

This Theory and Sleep Research Data

Has the view of function as we have outlined it accounted for the various striking facts about sleep which we have previously said should be explained by a theory of function? The major fact of the existence of two states of sleep and their temporal relation is encompassed by this theory, since I have suggested separate functions for S and D, but functions which are related in such a way that S, responsible for anabolism and production of macromolecules, must precede D, which may make use of some of these macromolecules in processes of restoration and reconnection.

The length of time occupied by S- and D-periods and by the cycle is roughly the amount of time that might be involved in macromolecule synthesis and in structural change. It is of course possible that what occurs during S and D are certain crucial steps in synthesis and structural change rather than the entire process; so that we can only say that the time intervals are at least compatible.

The views presented are compatible with the phylogenetic aspects of the states of sleep, since presumably it is only in the "higher" forms, especially mammals, that the cortical and corticopetal connections involving flexible guidance systems and so on can be assumed to exist. The ability to "repro-gram" oneself during life is certainly developed to the greatest extent, if not uniquely, in mammals. It must be admitted that within the class mammalia there are no clear differences in amount of D-time per 24 hours that can be related to complexity or flexibility of the particular species. It is hard to know what to make of this evidence, however, since a species with higher and more developed cortical systems may, on the one hand, require more of the restoration provided by sleep but, on the other hand, perhaps may be able to obtain this restoration more efficiently per minute of time. Certainly within our own species the changes produced by mental deficiency and senile dementia are very consistent with the views presented here.

The present theory is also compatible with the ontogeny of the sleep states, since a young animal or human obviously does more learning in a day, probably has more stress, and certainly has more reprogramming and rearranging of his central nervous system mechanisms than does an older individual.

Finally, the higher levels of cortical and forebrain arousal during D are compatible with these views, since times of increased memory consolidation and learning have always been associated with high cortical arousal levels.

Implications for Future Studies

It might also be worth considering whether this theory, in addition to accounting for present evidence, leads to any specific formulations for future studies and whether it could predict results of studies in progress. A number of suggested studies have already been mentioned, including studies of enzymes in the catecholamine synthetic pathway and electron microscope studies of cortical synapses.

One additional prediction from the theory presented here would be that inhibitors of macromolecule or protein synthesis would grossly interfere with the functions of both S- and D-sleep. One would certainly predict interference with the restorative properties of sleep in terms of mood, behavior, memory, and so on; it is difficult to predict specific effects on the organization of sleep, but one might well expect some alteration. Two preliminary reports on effects of protein synthesis inhibitors have so far produced conflicting results.[2]

This theory also has implications for the proliferating studies of D-deprivation and slow-wave sleep deprivation. Since it is postulated that the restorative functions attributed to D depend on proteins or other materials being made available during previous slow-wave sleep periods, one would expect that "D-deprivation effects," insofar as these can be identified, might result from slow-wave sleep deprivation as well as from D-deprivation; thus the conditions would be

2. Pegram, Hammond, and Bridgers 1972; Stern, Morgane, Panksepp, Zolovick, and Jalowiec 1972.

difficult to separate. From this point of view an appropriate control for D-deprivation would definitely not be slow-wave sleep deprivation or stage-4 deprivation, but perhaps awakenings during stage 2 spaced late during the night at approximately the same times as D-deprivation awakenings. However, specific studies of effects of slow-wave sleep deprivation are still possible. The restorative functions of slow-wave sleep are postulated to precede those of D-sleep, so that if appropriate tests were devised for the "physical" restoration produced by slow-wave sleep, defects should be found after slow-wave sleep deprivation but not after D-deprivation.[3]

3. I cannot resist noting that although sleep research appears to have come a long way, the functions I am proposing for the two states of sleep could be considered as merely adding precision to Shakespeare's formulation cited previously. Thus:
Let S—"chief nourisher at life's feast"—prepare
For D, "that knits up the raveled sleave of care."

14 Implications: The Chemistry of the Mind and Mind-Brain Relationships

I have now said all I can say about the functions of sleep. What follows can be considered an appendix or a speculative flight, but it may well also be the most important part of the book. Based partly on the discussion of sleep we have just completed, I should like first to develop briefly some hypotheses about the chemistry of the mind—specifically the role of the catecholamines in mental functioning. Then I shall end by presenting a framework for studying mind-brain relationships which I consider useful and probably necessary for works such as the present one.

Functions of the Catecholamines

The formulation I have arrived at—that sleep and especially D-sleep may have a role in restoring and reorganizing certain ascending catecholamine-containing systems and cortical networks influenced by these systems—leads to the obvious question of precisely what function these systems have during waking life. Animal studies have demonstrated several specific roles for brain catecholamines including feeding and satiety mechanisms in the hypothalamus and control of motor activity in the corpus striatum. I shall be more concerned here with possible roles in "higher" mental function, and these have been explored to a certain extent in previous chapters.

The catecholamines obviously play an important part in the higher functions of the brain. I have been extremely impressed clinically by the ability of a simple chemical—dextroamphetamine[1]—to produce a state of increased energy

1. As discussed previously, the amphetamines almost certainly act by releasing brain catecholamines and preventing their reuptake into cells—thus increasing synaptic availability of the catecholamines.

sometimes resembling hypomania when first administered, occasionally extreme compulsivity if too much is taken, a very definite paranoid state on continued administration of high doses, and a severe clinical depression after discontinuation. All these psychological states can be produced by alterations in brain catecholamine functioning in relatively normal individuals; attempts to explain these effects purely on the basis of predisposition to illness have not been successful. I would suggest that perhaps hypomania and compulsivity are induced by excessive amounts of dopamine or norepinephrine or stimulation of receptors in different specific areas; paranoia, by an excessive release such that dopamine receptors are stimulated far more than norepinephrine receptors (the amines may be released before norepinephrine is synthesized from dopamine); and depression after withdrawal, by a severe relative shortage of norepinephrine or dopamine (probably norepinephrine), only small or normal amounts being available when receptors have become used to overstimulation by the drug-induced release. This of course is a rough and oversimplified outline.

My concern here is not so much with the chemistry of psychiatric illness per se but with the chemistry of psychological concepts which are generally used to describe what goes on in the "mind" or "psyche." I suggest that certain psychoanalytic concepts are important shorthand expressions for complex brain processes which we can now begin to specify. I want to discuss specifically the possibility that certain facets of mental functioning so far explained rather well (though in a fashion hard to quantify or objectify) in psychological terms will turn out to be restatable in terms relating to the function of brain catecholamine systems. Elaborating on what has been suggested in chapters 12 and 13, I suggest that the important psychoanalytic concept of primary process refers to the functioning of the brain without the usual (waking) catecholamine influences from the ascending pathways we are considering[2] and that this is the situation

2. In anatomical terms, the systems I have been speaking about can best be

during D-sleep and perhaps during acute psychosis. Secondary process refers to the normal or alert waking functioning of these systems. In other words, I suggest that the ascending norepinephrine-containing systems are essential for the smooth balanced secondary-process functioning of waking.

Primary and secondary process are not the only psychological concepts which can probably be related to catecholamine systems. Thus, well-rested waking functioning, which I suggest involves normal functioning of these catecholamine systems, can be characterized psychoanalytically as relative ego autonomy from the drives and from the environment and optimal functioning of reality testing and other adaptive ego mechanisms. Tiredness, involving the wearing out of these adaptive ego mechanisms, less reality testing, and less ego autonomy, describes a state of poor functioning of these brain systems. These formulations are obviously compatible with other findings we have reviewed earlier, indicating that catecholamine systems may be involved in new learning, in optimistic or euphoric mood, in reward systems, and perhaps specifically in focused attention during wakefulness.

I have tried above to formulate the "higher" functions of the catecholamine systems (or catecholamine influences on the cerebral cortex) directly in psychoanalytic terms. I shall now also formulate these functions in somewhat different but related psychological terms which make most sense to me at present and which I have used at times throughout this book. I believe catecholamine influences may be involved in waking functions on three different levels: first, flexible focused attention—this refers to the perception of the world necessary for orienting oneself, an ability to concentrate on items of interest, to exclude others temporarily, and when necessary to shift the focus; then, on a broader level, patterning of the

related to the "dorsal norepinephrine bundle" described by the Karolinska Institute group (Anden, Dahlstrom, Fuxe, and Larsson 1965; Anden, Dahlstrom, Fuxe, Larsson, Olson, and Ungerstedt 1966).

environment—seeing patterns in one's surroundings and learning from them (not only recognizing but also testing and imposing patterns); and, still more broadly, feedback-modulated internal guidance systems—reacting to various stimuli from the environment, producing a series of homeostatic changes, and making the appropriate adjustments to allow the organism to proceed toward some eventual goal.[3] In the broadest sense I am now talking of flexible adaptation to the environment, social as well as purely physical. It is exactly these subtle feedback guidance systems, especially characteristic of mammalian waking brain function, which I have suggested wear out somewhat during tiredness and may be completely shunted out for repairs during D-sleep.

The catecholamine-mediated functions can be exaggerated, either in certain psychological conditions or as a result of overdose of amphetamines. Thus an overuse or exaggeration of the focusing mechanism can produce a compulsive character style or the well-known "riveted attention" found after high doses of amphetamines. The exaggeration of the patterning function is excessive pattern imposition, an insistence on finding patterns or meanings in the environment, as seen in the cognitive style characteristic of paranoia. Users of large repeated doses of amphetamines almost inevitably develop paranoia, and Ellinwood (1971) has demonstrated a somewhat similar development in monkeys and other species—an intense concentration followed by a determined looking under things (suspiciousness). And expert pattern imposers, for instance the greatest chess masters or masters at games such as building financial empires, frequently are at least a little paranoid.

Since this proposal suggests a very broad function for the catecholamines in promoting normal adaptive psychological functioning, it is obvious that malfunctioning of such a

3. Of course smooth, effective guidance directly involves realistic patterning, which in turn implies proper flexible focused attention mechanisms. Guidance describes the process at the highest level.

system could result in a variety of serious disturbances. We have touched above on some of the simpler possibilities involving excessive use or stimulation; and, previously, in discussing tiredness and sleep deprivation (also D-deprivation) we explored some effects of "depletion." Indeed, researchers working independently on various clinical problems without using any general formulations such as I am proposing have suggested that catecholamine dysfunction may play a role in mania and depression;[4] schizophrenia (Cohen, Allen, Pollin, and Hrubec 1972), especially paranoid schizophrenia (Ellinwood and Sudilovsky 1973); minimal brain dysfunction ("hyperkinetic syndrome") in children;[5] and compulsive tics (Meyerhoff and Snyder 1972). All this might involve the ascending norepinephrine bundles; I have not included here Parkinson's disease, tardive dyskinesia, and similar movement disorders probably related to nigrostriatal dopamine systems.

How could the ascending catecholamine systems do all this? It is possible that they exert some modulatory effect on the cortex quite apart from their synaptic neurotransmitter action; however, even considering simple synaptic activity in sheets of small neurons, as in the cortex, one might tentatively visualize a role for these amines in terms of producing clearly demarcated small areas of excitation surrounded by inhibition; "inhibitory sharpening" would be a possible description. In other words, smooth clear lines separating small areas of excitation from the surrounding inhibition would characterize a state of carefully balanced waking feedback homeostasis, while blurred lines leading to "spillover" of excitation would characterize less balanced, less delicately adjusted cortical functions such as I have suggested occur in tiredness or during dreaming. This inhibitory sharpening may underlie focused attention and exclusion of unwanted stimuli, which

4. Schildkraut, Schanberg, Breese, and Kopin 1967; Strom-Olsen and Weil-Malherbe 1958.

5. Arnold, Wender, McCloskey, and Snyder 1972; Wender 1971.

could on higher levels help to build a patterned, testable view of the environment and eventually allow the subtle physical and social feedback needed for guidance. These are exactly the functions which I have tried to show may wear out during a long day of wakefulness and need to be restored by sleep. And they are the same functions which are not found during dreaming sleep.

Mind-Brain Relationships

I have suggested above that certain psychological and psychoanalytic terms may refer to the functions of specifiable catecholamine-containing brain systems. Obviously the implication is that other such terms may well refer to other brain systems; and, in fact, I consider it likely that all useful psychological concepts which attempt to describe what goes on in the mind will eventually turn out to be shorthand descriptions of complex brain events. I shall amplify and discuss here a framework for examining these relationships, a framework I consider important or even essential for works such as this, in which one problem (such as the functions of sleep) is considered from various chemical, physiological, and psychoanalytic viewpoints.

The framework I am suggesting is diagrammed in figure 16 and is very similar to what I have discussed elsewhere (Hartmann 1968c). For simplicity's sake I suggest that we look first at a single moment in time and ask exactly what is going on in a person at that moment. At any moment during waking the person is having certain conscious subjective experiences including perceptions and feelings. This subjective experience is of great interest—it constitutes our entire world of experience—but the subjective experience cannot be studied directly by science, and its "essence" is perhaps never entirely ascertainable.[6] Yet, as I have suggested (1968c; and

6. This is the old question of whether two persons actually have the same experience when each sees a green object. They could be having very

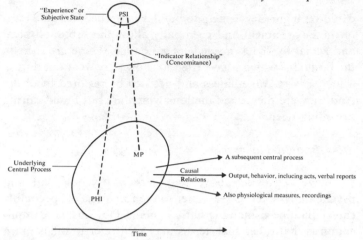

Figure 16. A framework for looking at events in the mind. PSI states (subjective states, feelings, etc.) cannot be studied directly. They are useful as concomitants or indicators of underlying processes—what is really going on at a given moment—which can be described in terms of brain events (PHI) or in terms of the "metapsychological" (MP) concepts of psychoanalytic terminology. Useful MP-state concepts will probably turn out to be shorthand for PHI states.

see chapter 12), the experience can be used scientifically as a concomitant or indicator of the underlying process or central state.

It is the underlying process which can be studied directly, and approaches to it can be made from a variety of directions. The neurophysiologist or chemist can approach the underlying process at any given moment by examining tracings or displays of physiological events almost simultaneously—a few milliseconds or seconds afterward—or he can examine changes in peripheral physiology or in blood or urine for a longer time thereafter. From all this he can arrive at some formulation of the person's central state or underlying processes in physiological or chemical terms. Needless to

different subjective sensations without the least disagreement between them about which objects are called "green." Similarly, are two persons experiencing the same thing when they say they feel happy or sad?

say, at the present stage of our knowledge his formulation must be extremely incomplete, even if it represents data from thousands of individual neurons, neuronal systems, or chemical outputs.

The observer of behavior, especially the trained psychological observer or psychoanalyst, can approach the underlying process by examining behavior, including the person's actions or nonverbal behavior and also his verbal reports of actions and of experiences or feelings. Using these behaviors and reports, and his previous knowledge of the person, the analyst can then try to formulate what was going on (underlying process) in terms of the person's ego, his defenses against drives, his coping mechanisms, the distribution of his "psychic energy," and so on. The formulations of the psychoanalyst will be less quantitative and objective (in the sense that the observations are far less easy for observers to report and to agree upon) than those of the physiologist, but they will be more ambitious in the sense of an attempt at a total description.

The important point as I see it is that both scientists are studying *the same thing*. Although one group of terms used may derive historically from electrical studies of a giant squid axon, and another group of terms may derive from hours spent listening to a neurotic Viennese patient, and others from yet other sources, they are all attempting to describe the same entity, the underlying process, or "what is really going on" in a person at a given moment.

The central state at a given moment has been discussed for the sake of simplicity, but obviously I believe that the same arguments are true when central processes lasting over time are considered. There is no mysterious leap or mind-body gap between the physiological-chemical description and the psychological description of the underlying process or central state.[7] The "gap" or "leap" exists only between the subjective

7. Psychoanalysts have used the word *metapsychological* to refer to their psychological concepts, but this has the unfortunate connotation (metaphys-

experience (also called "psychic experience" or "PSI-state") and the underlying process (see figure 16).

In this sense the ego *is* the brain, with the emphasis on the verb *is,* rather than on the nouns. I do not wish to argue about the exact boundaries of the ego or the brain—the superego of course would have to be included also—but rather to emphasize the identity of what is being described— the totality of the underlying central processes responsible for perception, for handling and channeling whatever energy is available, for directing the motor activity of the organism. Both the ego and the brain have been referred to, in separate contexts, as the "organ of adaptation."

As it stands, the statement of identity (ego is brain) can serve as a conceptual frame but is too broad to be of direct scientific use. Also, certain obvious specific derivatives (looking at small aspects of ego function and brain function) have not usually been fruitful. For instance, there is no doubt in my mind that a complex cognitive process such as that which occurs when a person learns a new language must be associated with changes in the brain. I am equally certain, however, that such changes are on a level too subtle to be worth discussing neurologically or neurochemically at present. However, I believe that many of the concepts dealt with by psychiatry and psychoanalysis are on a much larger, grosser level, where it does already make sense to examine and conceptualize the same processes from the two starting points. And I have suggested above that certain specific psychological concepts (secondary process) may be describing the same process as certain neurochemical formulations (normal waking functioning of the cortex under the influence of ascending catecholamine pathways). In such areas I believe the framework can be of immediate use.

Since I have occasionally resorted to the use of computer

ics) of "beyond" real psychology (thus "far out"). This had historical justification, but it now seems essential to emphasize that these terms, as well as others derived from other disciplines interested in underlying process, *are* psychology.

terms throughout this book, let me formulate the identity in another way and say that ego-terms may be a higher-level language, specifying exactly the same programs and operations that can be specified (in greater detail but necessarily at much greater length) in the lower-level language of neurophysiology and chemistry.

All this has obvious implications for the study of the human mind. A huge discipline-imposed gap has grown where a clear look reveals that no actual gap exists. The neurophysiologist or other neuro-scientist (and this includes the physiological psychologist and the biopsychologist) pursues his work carefully without paying much attention to the "mind" or ego concepts for which the work may be relevant. At the end of a long empirical paper he may occasionally suggest that his work may have implications for "higher" functions; but these are likely to be at most something like "sensory integration" or "reward or punishment systems." He considers that terms such as *ego defenses* or *secondary process* are either nonsense or vague generalizations of little concern to him. He may of course be entirely right in sticking to his work and refusing to become involved in hard-to-define psychological terms, but I would suggest that he is nonetheless studying these concepts or at least providing some of the blocks of which they are built. It might even at times be useful for him to be aware of them not in terms of influencing the day-to-day nature of his work, but possibly in helping him decide, when he is at some "branch point" in his work, what general directions could be of most interest and importance in the total understanding of man.

In general the psychiatrist or psychoanalyst, although his theory includes important building blocks for a psychology of the mind, has been satisfied with a purely clinical vantage point from which terms such as ego or primary process are seen as somewhat distant distillations, derived from direct work with patients. I would agree that indeed what he says of these terms is true, but this describes their historical derivation, not their place in the study of the mind. The psychoanalyst tends to consider the brain as a lump of tissue perhaps examined long ago in medical school and now studied only by an assorted group of neuro-scientists who may be competent in their specialities but understand little of the "true" (i.e. psychodynamic) workings of the human mind. He may even say something like "the ego is a concept; the brain is an organ," as if that disposed of the problem. Surely, it would be useful to him to notice that perhaps some of the concepts he deals with do not have to be "left floating" (Freud's term) but may very well be shorthand descriptions, or descriptions in a higher order language, of an underlying process which could also be specified in terms of the brain.

What I am saying is that in spite of ourselves and the limitations of our disciplines, we are studying the same thing—the human mind; and I have suggested some specific examples where this identity may already be visible and useful. It is perhaps ironic that the field I have been discussing is obviously *psychology*—the study of the mind— yet the present discipline of psychology has hardly entered into the discussion. Although there are individual psychologists who are intensely involved in both the neuro-sciences and the clinical psychoanalytic aspects, behaviorism—the dominant school of American psychology—has, for various historical reasons, not concerned itself at all with underlying process or central state; thus although it has produced many important advances in the understanding and control of behavior, it has avoided the central issue of psychology as I see it. Perhaps it is time for a new psychology, based on concepts from the neuro-sciences and from psychoanalysis or other psychologies, which does approach and attempt to formulate the problems of underlying process. The present work has suggested some possible beginnings along such lines.

Bibliography

Adey, W. R. 1966. Neurophysiological correlates of information transaction and storage in brain tissue. In *Progress in Physiological Psychology,* E. Stellar and J. M. Sprague, eds., vol. 1, pp. 1–43. New York: Acad. Pr.

Adey, W. R.; Bores, E.; and Porter, R. 1968. EEG sleep patterns after high cervical lesions in man. *Arch. Neurol.* 19:377–83.

Agnew, H. W., Jr.; Webb, W. B.; and Williams, R. L. 1964. The effects of stage four sleep deprivation. *Electroencephalog. Clin. Neurophysiol.* 17:68–70.

Agnew, H. W., Jr.; Webb, W. B.; and Williams, R. L. 1967. Comparison of stage four and 1-REM sleep deprivation. *Percept. Motor Skills* 24:851–58.

Akindele, M. O.; Evans, J. I.; and Oswald, I. 1970. Mono-Amine oxidase inhibitors, sleep and mood. *Electroencephalog. Clin. Neurophysiol.* 29:47–56.

Albert, I.; Cicala, G. A.; and Siegal, J. 1970. The behavioral effects of REM sleep deprivation in rats. *Psychophysiology* 6:550–60.

Allen, S.; Oswald, I.; and Tagney, J. 1971. The effects of distorted visual input on sleep. Report to the 1st International Congress of the Association for the Psychophysiological Study of Sleep, June, Bruges, Belgium.

Allison, T.; Van Twyver, G.; and Goff, W. R. 1972. Electrophysiological studies of the echidna, *Tachyglossus aculeatus.* 1. Waking and sleep. *Arch. Ital. Biol.* 110:145–84.

Anden, N. E.; Dahlstrom, A.; Fuxe, K.; and Larsson, K. 1965. Mapping out of catecholamine and 5-hydroxytryptamine neurons innervating the telencephalon and diencephalon. *Life Sciences* 4:1275–79.

Anden, N. E.; Dahlstrom, A.; Fuxe, K.; Larsson, K.; Olson, L.; and Ungerstedt, U. 1966. Ascending monoamine neurons to the telencephalon and diencephalon. *Acta Physiol. Scand.* 67:313–26.

Armington, J. C., and Mitnick, L. L. 1959. Electroencephalogram and sleep deprivation. *J. Appl. Physiol.* 14:247–50.

Arnold, L. E.; Wender, P. H.; McCloskey, K.; and Snyder, S. H. 1972. Levoamphetamine and dextroamphetamine: comparative efficacy in the hyperkinetic syndrome. *Arch. Gen. Psychiat.* 27:816–22.

Aserinsky, E., and Kleitman, N. 1953. Regularly occurring periods of eye motility and concomitant phenomena during sleep. *Science* 118:273–74.

Aserinsky, E., and Kleitman, N. 1955. Two types of ocular motility occurring in sleep. *J. Appl. Physiol.* 8:1–10.

Astic, L., and Jouvet-Monnier, D. 1970. Etude in utero des etats de veille et de sommeil chez le cobaye. *J. Physiol.* 62(suppl.):115–16.

Ax, A., and Luby, E. D. 1961. Autonomic responses to sleep deprivation. *Arch. Gen. Psychiat.* 4:55–59.

Baekeland, F. 1970. Exercise and deprivation: sleep and psychological reactions. *Arch. Gen. Psychiat.* 22:365–69.

Baekeland, F., and Hartmann, E. 1970. Sleep requirements and the characteristics of some sleepers. In *Sleep and Dreaming*, ed. E. Hartmann, pp. 33–43. International Psychiatry Clinics Series, vol. 7. Boston: Little, Brown.

Baekeland, F., and Hartmann, E. 1971. Reported sleep characteristics: effects of age, sleep length and psychiatric impairment. *Comp. Psychiat.* 12:141–47.

Baekeland, F., and Lasky, R. 1966. Exercise and sleep patterns in college athletes. *Percept. Motor Skills* 23:1203–07.

Baekeland, F., and Lundwall, L. 1971. Effects of methyldopa on sleep patterns in man. *Electroencephalog. Clin. Neurophysiol.* 31:269–73.

Bartley, S. H. 1965. *Fatigue: Mechanism and Management.* Springfield, Ill.: Charles C. Thomas.

Bast, T. H. 1925. Morphological changes in fatigue. *Wisc. Med. J.* 24:271–72.

Benoit, O., and Bloch, V. 1960. Seuil d'excitabilite reticulaire et sommeil profond chez le chat. *J. Physiol.* 52:17–18.

Berger, R. J. 1969. Oculomotor control: a possible function of REM sleep. *Psychol. Rev.* 76:144–64.

Berger, R., and Oswald, I. 1962. Effects of sleep deprivation on behavior, subsequent sleep, and dreaming. *J. Ment. Sci.* 108:457–65.

Blake, H., and Gerard, R. W. 1937. Brain potentials during sleep. *Amer. J. Physiol.* 119:692–703.

Bliss, E. L.; Clark, L. D.; and West, C. D. 1959. Studies of sleep deprivation: relationship to schizophrenia. *Arch. Neurol. Psychiat.* 81:348–59.

Bloom, F. E.; Algeri, S.; Groppetti, A.; Revuelta, A.; and Costa, A. 1969. Lesions of central norepinephrine terminals with 6-OH-dopamine: biochemistry and fine structure. *Science* 166:1284–86.

Boland, B. D., and Dewsbury, D. A. 1971. Characteristics of sleep following sexual activity and wheel running in male rats. *Physiol. Behav.* 6:145–49.

Breger, L. 1967. Functions of dreams. *J. Abnorm. Psychol.* Monograph no. 641.

Breger, L.; Hunter, I.; and Lane, R. W. 1971. The effects of stress on dreams. *Psychological Issues.* Monograph no. 27. New York: Intl. Univs. Pr.

Brewer, V., and Hartmann, E. 1973. Variable sleepers: when is more or less sleep required. Report to the Association for the Psychophysiological Study of Sleep, San Diego.

Brill, R. W., and Goodman, I. J. 1969. Effects of REM sleep deprivation on memory in cats. *Psychophysiol.* 6:226.

Brooks, D., and Bizzi, E. 1963. Brain stem electrical activity during sleep. *Arch. Ital. Biol.* 101:648–65.

Cadilhac, J.; Passouant-Fontaine, T.; and Passouant, P. 1961. Modifications de l'activite de l'hippocampe suivant les divers stades du sommeil spontane chez le chat. *Rev. Neurol.* 105:171–76.

Cadilhac, J.; Passouant-Fontaine, T.; and Passouant, P. 1962. L'organisation des divers stades du sommeil chez le chaton, de la naissance à 45 jours. *J. Physiol.* 54:305–06.

Callaway, E., and Dembo, D. 1958. Narrowed attention. *Arch. Neurol. Psychiat.* 79:74–90.

Callaway, E., and Thompson, S. 1953. Sympathetic activity and perception. *Psychosom. Med.* 15:443–45.

Carr, L., and Moore, K. 1969. Norepinephrine: release from brain by d-amphetamine *in vivo. Science* 164:322–23.

Chernick, D. A. 1972. Effect of REM sleep deprivation on learning and recall by humans. *Percept. Motor Skills* 34:283–94.

Claparède, E. 1908. La fonchon du sommeil. *Revista di Scienza* 2:141–58.

Cohen, H., and Dement, W. 1965. Sleep: changes in threshold to electroconvulsive shock in rats after deprivation of paradoxical phase. *Science* 150:1318–19.

Cohen, H., and Dement, W. 1966. Sleep: suppression of rapid eye movement phase in the cat after electroconvulsive shock. *Science* 154:396–98.

Cohen, S. M.; Allen, M. G.; Pollin, W.; and Hrubec, Z. 1972. Relationship of schizo-affective psychosis to manic depressive psychosis and schizophrenia. *Arch. Gen. Psychiat.* 26:539–46.

Cordeau, J. P.; De Champlain, J.; and Jacks, B. 1971. Excitation and prolonged waking produced by catecholamines injected into the ventricular system of cats. *Canad. J. Physiol. Pharmacol.* 49:627–31.

Coriat, I. H. 1912. The nature of sleep. *J. Abnorm. Psychol.* 6:329–67.

Cramer, H., and Kuhlo, W. 1967. Effets des inhibiteurs de la monoaminoxidase sur le sommeil et l'electroencephalogramme chez l'homme. *Acta Neurol. Belg.* 67:658–69.

Cuny, H. 1962. *Ivan Pavlov, the Man and His Theories.* New York: Fawcett World.

Dement, W. 1960. The effect of dream deprivation. *Science* 131: 1705–07.

Dement, W. 1964. Experimental dream studies. In *Science and Psychoanalysis: Scientific Proceedings of the Academy of Psychoanalysis*, ed. J. Masserman, vol. 7, pp. 129–62. New York: Grune.

Dement, W. 1965. Recent studies on the biological role of rapid eye movement sleep. *Amer. J. Psychiat.* 122:404–08.

Dement, W. 1970. The biological role of REM sleep (ca. 1968). In *Sleep: Physiology and Pathology, A Symposium*, ed. A. Kales, pp. 245–65. Philadelphia: Lippincott.

Dement, W.; Ferguson, F.; Cohen, H.; and Barchas, J. 1969. Nonchemical methods and data using a biochemical model: the REM quanta. In *Psychochemical Research in Man*, ed. A. J. Mandell and M. P. Mandell, pp. 275–325. New York: Acad. Pr.

Dement, W.; Henry, P.; Cohen, H.; and Ferguson, J. 1967. Studies on the effect of REM deprivation in humans and in animals. *Research Publications Association Research in Nervous and Mental Disease* 45:456–68.

Dement, W., and Wolpert, E. 1958. Relation of eye movements, body motility, and external stimuli to dream content. *J. Exp. Psychol.* 55:543–53.

Dement, W.; Zarcone, V.; Ferguson, J.; Cohen, H.; Pivik, T.; and Barchas, J. 1969. Some parallel findings in schizophrenic patients and serotonin-depleted cats. In *Schizophrenia: Current Concepts and Research*, ed. D. B. Siva Sankar, pp. 775–811. Hicksville, N.Y.: PJD Publications.

Detre, T.; Himmelhoch, J.; Swartzburg, M.; Anderson, C. M.; Byck,

R.; and Kupfer, D. J. 1972. Hypersomnia and manic-depressive disease. *Amer. J. Psychiat.* 128:1303–05.

Dewan, E. M. 1969. The programming "P" hypothesis. *Physical Sciences Paper* no. 388, AFCRL-69-0298, July.

Dewan, E. M. 1970. The programming "P" hypothesis for REM sleep. In *Sleep and Dreaming*, ed. E. Hartmann, International Psychiatry Clinics Series, vol. 7, pp. 295–307. Boston: Little, Brown.

Dewson, J.; Dement, W.; Wagener, T.; and Nobel, K. 1967. Rapid eye movement sleep deprivation: a central-neural change during wakefulness. *Science* 156:403–06.

Dillon, R. F., and Webb, W. B. 1965. Threshold of arousal from "activated" sleep in the rat. *J. Comp. Physiol. Psychol.* 59:446–47.

Dodge, R. 1917. The loss of relative fatigue. *Psychol. Rev.* 24:89–113.

Doty, B., and Doty, L. 1966. Facilitation effects of amphetamine avoidance conditioning in relation to age and problem difficulty. *Psychopharmacologia* 9:234–41.

Dunleavy, D. L. F., and Oswald, I. 1972. Sleep and thyrotoxicosis. Report to the 11th Annual Meeting of the Association for the Psychophysiological Study of Sleep, May, Lake Minnewaska, New York. In *Sleep Research 1971–1972*, ed. M. Chase, W. C. Stern, and P. Walter. Los Angeles: Brain Information Service, UCLA.

Ellinwood, E. H. 1971. Comparative metamphetamine intoxication in experimental animals. *Pharmakospsychiat. Neuro-psychopharm.* 4:351–61.

Ellinwood, E. H., and Sudilovsky, A. 1973. Chronic amphetamine intoxication: behavioral model of psychoses. Unpublished studies.

Ephron, H. S., and Carrington, P. 1966. Rapid eye movement sleep and cortical homeostasis. *Psychol. Rev.* 73:500–26.

Evans, W. O., and Smith, R. P. 1964. Some effects of morphine and amphetamine on intellectual functions and mood. *Psychopharmacologia* 6:49.

Evarts, E. 1962. Activity of neurons in visual cortex of cat during sleep with low voltage fast EEG activity. *J. Neurophysiol.* 25:812–16.

Evarts, E. 1967. Unit activity in sleep and wakefulness. In *The Neurosciences: A Study Program*, ed. G. C. Quarton, T. Melnechuk, and F. O. Schmitt, pp. 545–56. New York: Rockefeller.

Feinberg, I. 1968a. The ontogenesis of human sleep and the relationship of sleep variables to intellectual function in the aged. *Comp. Psychiat.* 9:138–47.

Feinberg, I. 1968*b*. Eye movement activity during sleep and intellectual function in mental retardation. *Science* 159:1256.

Feinberg, I., and Carlson, V. R. 1968. Sleep variables as a function of age in man. *Arch. Gen. Psychiat.* 18:239–50.

Feinberg, I., and Evarts, E. 1969*a*. Changing concepts of the function of sleep: discovery of intense brain activity during sleep calls for revision of hypotheses as to its function. *Biol. Psychiat.* 1:331–48.

Feinberg, I., and Evarts, E. 1969*b*. Some implications of sleep research for psychiatry. In *Neurobiological Aspects of Psychopathology*, Proc. Amer. Psychopath. Ass. 58:334–93. New York: Grune.

Feinberg, I.; Koresko, R. L.; Heller, N.; and Steinberg, H. R. 1966. Sleep EEG and eye-movement patterns in young and aged normal subjects and in patients with chronic brain syndrome. Paper read at the 4th World Congress of Psychiatry, Sept. 5–10, 1966, Madrid, Spain.

Fencl, V.; Koski, G.; and Pappenheimer, J. R. 1971. Factors in cerebrospinal fluid from goats that affect sleep and activity in rats. *J. Physiol.* 216:565–89.

Ferguson, J., and Dement, W. 1967. The effect of REM sleep deprivation on the lethality of dextroamphetamine sulfate in grouped rats. *Psychophysiology* 4:380.

Fishbein, W. 1971. Disruptive effects of rapid eye movement sleep deprivation on long-term memory. *Physiol. Behav.* 6:279–82.

Fishbein, W.; McGaugh, J. L.; and Swarz, J. R. 1971. Retrograde amnesia: electroconvulsive shock effects after termination of rapid eye movement sleep deprivation. *Science* 172:80–82.

Fisher, C. 1965*a*. Psychoanalytic implications of recent research on sleep and dreaming. I. Empirical findings. *J. Amer. Psychoanal. Ass.* 13:1927–70.

Fisher, C. 1965*b*. Psychoanalytic implications of recent research on sleep and dreaming. II. Implications of psychoanalytic theory. *J. Amer. Psychonal. Ass.* 13:271–303.

Fisher, C. 1966. Dreaming and sexuality. In *Psychoanalysis: A General Psychology*, ed. R. Lowenstein, L. Newman, M. Schur, and A. Solnit, pp. 537–69. New York: Intl. Univs. Pr.

Fisher, C.; Gross, J.; and Zuch, J. 1965. Cycle of penile erection synchronous with dreaming (REM) sleep, a preliminary report. *Arch. Gen. Psychiat.* 12:29–45.

Foulkes, D. 1966. *The Psychology of Sleep.* New York: Scribner.

Frederickson, C. J., and Hobson, J. A. 1969. The sleep of cats following prolonged electrical stimulation of the brain stem reticular activating system. *Psychophysiology* 6:271.

Freemon, F. R. 1970. Reciprocal environmental surveillance model of sleep. *J. Theor. Biol.* 27:339–40.

Freemon, F. R. 1972. *Sleep Research: A Critical Review.* Springfield, Ill.: Charles C. Thomas.

French, T. M., and Fromm, E. 1964. *Dream Interpretation: A New Approach.* New York: Basic Books.

Freud, S. 1953. Interpretation of dreams. In *Standard Edition of the Complete Psychological Works of Sigmund Freud*, ed. J. Strachey, vol. 4 (of 24 Volumes). London: Hogarth.

Fuxe, K.; Hokfelt, T.; and Ungerstedt, U. 1971. Morphological and functional aspects of central monoamine neurons. *Int. Rev. Neurobiol.* 13:93–126.

Gaarder, K. 1966. A conceptual model of sleep. *Arch. Gen. Psychiat.* 14:253–60.

Garma, A. 1966. *The Psychoanalysis of Dreams.* New York: Dell.

Glowinski, J., and Axelrod, J. 1965. Effects of drugs on the uptake, release, and metabolism of the H^3-norepinephrine in rat brain. *J. Pharmacol. Exp. Ther.* 149:43–49.

Greenberg, R., and Dewan, E. M. 1969. Aphasia and rapid eye movement sleep. *Nature* 223:183–84.

Greenberg R., and Leiderman, P. 1966. Perceptions, the dream process and memory: an up-to-date version of notes on a mystic writing pad. *Comp. Psychiat.* 7:517–22.

Greenberg, R.; Mayer, R.; Brook, R.; Pearlman, C.; and Hartmann, E. 1968. Sleep and dreaming in patients with post-alcoholic Korsakoff's disease. *Arch. Gen. Psychiat.* 18:203–09.

Greenberg, R., and Pearlman, C. 1972. REM sleep and the analytic process: a psycho-physiologic bridge. Report to the American Psychoanalytical Association, December, New York.

Greenberg, R.; Pearlman, C.; Fingar, R.; Kantrowitz, J.; and Kawliche, S. 1970. The effects of dream deprivation: implications for a theory of the psychological function of dreaming. *Brit. J. Med. Psychol.* 43:1–11.

Griffiths, W. J.; Lester, B. K.; Coulter, J. D.; and Williams, H. L. 1972. Tryptophan and sleep in young adults. *Psychophysiology* 9:345–56.

Haider, I., and Oswald, I. 1971. Effects of amylobarbitone and nitrazepam on the electrodermogram and other features. *Brit. J. Psychiat.* 118:519–22.

Hanson, L. 1967. Evidence that the central action of (+)-amphetamine is mediated via catecholamines. *Psychopharmacologia* 10:289–97.

Hartmann, E. 1966*a*. Dreaming sleep (the D-state) and the menstrual cycle. *J. Nerv. Ment. Dis.* 143:406–16.

Hartmann, E. 1966*b*. Reserpine: its effect on the sleep-dream cycle in man. *Psychopharmacologia* 9:242–47.

Hartmann, E. 1966*c*. The psychophysiology of free will. In *Psychoanalysis: A General Psychology*, ed. R. Lowenstein, L. Newman, M. Schur, and A. Solnit, pp. 521–36. New York: Intl. Univs. Pr.

Hartmann, E. 1967. *The Biology of Dreaming*. Springfield, Ill.: Charles C. Thomas.

Hartmann, E. 1968*a*. Longitudinal studies of sleep and dream patterns in manic-depressive patients. *Arch. Gen. Psychiat.* 19:312–29.

Hartmann, E. 1968*b*. The effect of four drugs on sleep in man. *Psychopharmacologia* 12:346–53.

Hartmann, E. 1969. Antidepressants and sleep: clinical and theoretical implications. In *Sleep Physiology and Pathology, A Symposium*, ed. A. Kales, pp. 308–16. Philadelphia: Lippincott.

Hartmann, E., ed. 1970*a*. Sleep and Dreaming. International Psychiatry Clinics Series vol. 7. Boston: Little, Brown.

Hartmann, E. 1970*b*. The D-state and norephinephrine-dependent systems. In *Sleep and Dreaming*, ed. E. Hartmann, International Psychiatry Clinics, vol. 7, pp. 308–28. Boston: Little, Brown.

Hartmann, E. 1970*c*. Pharmacology of dreaming sleep and its psychiatric implications. In *The Psychodynamic Implications of the Physiological Studies in Dreams*, ed. L. Madow, pp. 47–70. Springfield, Ill.: Charles C. Thomas.

Hartmann, E. 1971. L-tryptophane as a physiological hypnotic. *The Lancet* 1:807–08.

Hartmann, E. In press. Effect of psychotropic drugs on desynchronized sleep. In *Psychotropic Drugs and the Human EEG*, ed. T. M. Itil. Basel and New York: Karger.

Hartmann, E.; Baekeland, F.; Zwilling, G. 1972. Psychological differences between long and short sleepers. *Arch. Gen. Psychiat.* 26:463–68.

Hartmann, E.; Baekeland, F.; Zwilling, G.; and Hoy, P. 1971. Sleep need: How much sleep and what kind? *Amer. J. Psychiat.* 127:1001–08.

Hartmann, E., and Bridwell, T. J. 1970. Effects of AMPT, l-DOPA, and l-tryptophane on sleep in the rat. *Psychophysiology* 7:313.

Hartmann, E.; Bridwell, T. J.; and Schildkraut, J. J. 1971. Alpha-methylparatyrosine and sleep in the rat. *Psychopharmacologia* 21:157–64.

Hartmann, E.; Chung, R.; and Chien, C. 1971. L-tryptophane and sleep. *Psychopharmacologia* 19:114–27.

Hartmann, E.; Chung, R.; Draskoczy, P. R.; and Schildkraut, J. J. 1971. Effects of 6-hydroxydopamine on sleep in the rat. *Nature* 233:425–27.

Hartmann, E., and Cravens, J. To be published. Long-term drug effects on human sleep. *Psychopharmacologia.*

Hartmann, E.; Cravens, J.; Auchincloss, S.; Bernstein, J.; Beroz, M.; Marsden, H.; Stanford, G.; Sullivan, P.; and Wise, S. 1972. Placebo, reserpine, amitriptyline, chlorpromazine, chloral hydrate, and chlordiazepoxide: long-term effects on human sleep. Report to the 11th Annual Meeting of the Association for the Psychophysiological Study of Sleep, May, Lake Minnewaska, New York. Abstract in *Sleep Research 1971–1972,* ed. M. Chase, W. Stern, and P. Walter. Los Angeles: Brain Information Service, UCLA.

Hartmann, E.; Cravens, J.; and List, S. 1973. l-Tryptophane as a natural hypnotic: a dose response study in man. Report to the Association for the Psychophysiological Study of Sleep, May, San Diego.

Hartmann, E.; Galginaitis, C.; Moran, E.; Owen, A.; and Buchanan, K. 1972. When do we need more or less sleep: a study of variable sleepers. Report to the 11th Annual Meeting of the Association for the Psychophysiological Study of Sleep, May, Lake Minnewaska, New York. Abstract in *Sleep Research 1971–1972,* ed. M. Chase, W. Stern, and P. Walter. Los Angeles: Brain Information Service, UCLA.

Hartmann, E.; Marcus, J.; and Leinoff, A. 1968. The sleep-dream cycle and convulsion threshold. *Psychonom. Sci.* 13:141–42.

Hartmann, E., and Popper, C. 1972. Brain tyrosine hydroxylase: effects of D-deprivation and other forms of stress. Report to the 11th Annual Meeting of the Association for the Psychophysiological Study of Sleep. May, Lake Minnewaska, New York. Abstract in *Sleep Research 1971–1972,* ed. M. Chase, W. Stern, and P. Walter. Los Angeles: Brain Information Service, UCLA.

Hartmann, E., and Schildkraut, J. J. 1973. Desynchronized sleep and MHPG excretion: an inverse relationship. Report to the Association for the Psychophysiological Study of Sleep, May, San Diego.

Hartmann, E., and Stern, W. C. 1972. Desynchronized sleep deprivation: learning deficit and its reversal by increased catecholamines. *Physiol. Behav.* 8:585–87.

Hartmann, E.; Verdone, P.; and Snyder, F. 1966. Longitudinal studies of sleep and dreaming patterns in psychiatric patients. *J. Nerv. Ment. Dis.* 142:117–26.

Hartmann, E., and Wise, S. 1972. Unpublished studies.

Hartmann, E.; Zwilling, G. R.; and Chung, R. 1973. Unpublished studies.

Hartmann, E.; Zwilling, G. R.; and Koski, S. 1973. The effects of pimozide on sleep in the rat. Report to the Association for the Psychophysiological Study of Sleep, May, San Diego.

Hauri, P. 1968. Effects of evening activity on early night sleep. *Psychophysiology* 4:267–77.

Hawkins, D. R. 1966. A review of psychoanalytic dream theory in the light of recent psycho-physiological studies of sleep and dreaming. *Brit. J. Med.* 39:85–104.

Hennevin, E., and Leconte, P. 1971. La fonction du sommeil paradoxal: faits et hypotheses. *L'Ann. Psychologique* 2.

Herman, J.; Tauber, E.; Rosenman, C.; and Roffwarg, H. 1971. Stereopsis, state of sleep and visual input deprivation. Report to the 1st International Congress of the Association for the Psychophysiological Study of Sleep, June, Bruges, Belgium.

Hess, W. R. 1929. The mechanism of sleep. *Amer. J. Physiol.* 90:386–87.

Hess, W. R. 1931a. Le sommeil. *C. R. Soc. Biol.* 107:1333–64.

Hess, W. R. 1931b. On the interrelationships between psychic and vegetative function. *J. Nerv. Ment. Dis.* 74:511–28, 645–53.

Hess, W. R. 1965. Sleep as a phenomenon of the integral organism. In *Sleep Mechanisms*, ed. K. Akert, C. Bally, and J. P. Schade, pp. 3–8. Amsterdam: Elsevier.

Ho, M. A. 1972. Sex hormones and the sleep of women. Ph.D. Diss., Yeshiva University.

Hobson, J. A. 1968. Sleep after exercise. *Science* 162:1503–05.

Hobson, J. A., and Mc Carley, R. W. 1971. *Neuronal Activity in Sleep: an Annotated Bibliography.* Los Angeles: Brain Information Service, UCLA.

Hockey, G. R. 1970. Changes in attention allocation in a multicomponent task under loss of sleep. *Brit. J. Psychol.* 61:473–80.

Honda, Y.; Takahashi, K.: Takahashi, S.; Azumi, K.; Irie, M.; Sakuma, M.; Tsushima, T.; and Schizume, K. 1969. Growth hormone secretion during nocturnal sleep in normal subjects. *J. Clin. Endocrin.* 29:20–29.

Jackson, J. H. 1932. *Selected Writings of John Hughlings Jackson*, ed. J. Taylor. vols. 1, 2. London: Hodder and Stoughton.

Jacobson, A.; Kales, A.; Lehman, D.; and Hoedemacher, F. 1964. Muscle tonus in human subjects during sleep and dreaming. *Exp. Neurol.* 10:418–24.

Johnson, L. C.; Slye, E. S.; and Dement, W. 1965. Electroencephalograph and autonomic activity during and after prolonged sleep deprivation. *Psychosom. Med.* 27:415–22.

Jones, B. E. 1969. Catecholamine-containing neurons in the brain stem of the cat and their role in waking. These de Medecine, Univ. Lyon.

Jones, B. E.; Bobilier, P.; and Jouvet, M. 1969. Effets de la déstruction des neurones contenant des catécholamines du mésencephale sur le cycle veille-sommeils du chat. *C.R. Soc. Biol.* 163:176–80.

Jones, R. M. 1962. *Ego Synthesis in Dreams*. Cambridge, Mass.: Schenkman.

Jouvet, D.; Valatx, J.; and Jouvet, M. 1961. Etude polygraphique du sommeil du chaton. *C.R. Soc. Biol.* 155:1660–64.

Jouvet, M. 1961. Telencephalic and rhombencephalic sleep in the cat. In *CIBA Foundation Symposium on the Nature of Sleep*, ed. G. Wolstenholme and M. O'Connor. Boston: Little, Brown.

Jouvet, M. 1962. Récherches sur les structures neveuses et les mecanismes responsables des differentes phases du sommeil physiologique. *Arch. Ital. Biol.* 100:125–206.

Jouvet, M. 1969. Biogenic amines and the states of sleep. *Science* 163:32–41.

Jouvet, M., and Renault, J. 1966. Insomnie persistante après lesions des nouyaux du raphe chez le chat. *C.R. Soc. Biol.* 160:1461–65.

Jouvet, M.; Vimont, P.; and Delorme, F. 1965. Suppression élective du sommeil paradoxal chez le chat par les inhibiteurs de la monoamineoxidase. *C.R. Soc. Biol.* 159:1595.

Joy, R., and Prinz, P. 1969. The effect of sleep altering environments upon the acquisition and retention of a conditioned avoidance response in the rat. *Physiol. Behav.* 4:809–14.

Jus, A.; Jus, K.; Villeneuve, A.; Pires, A.; Fortier, J.; Lachance, R.; and Villeneuve, R. 1972. Studies on dream recall in chronic schizophrenic patients after frontal lobotomy. Report to the 11th Annual Meeting of the Association for the Psychophysiological Study of Sleep, May, Lake Minnewaska, New York. Abstract in *Sleep Research 1971–1972*, ed. M. Chase, W. Stern, and P. Walter. Los Angeles: Brain Information Service, UCLA.

Kales, A.; Allen, C.; Scharf, M. B.; and Kales, J. D. 1970. Hypnotic drugs and their effectiveness. *Arch. Gen. Psychiat.* 23:226–32.

Kales, A.; Heuser, G.; Jacobson, A.; Kales, J. D.; Hanley, J.; Zweizig, J. R.; and Paulson, M.J. 1967. All-night sleep patterns in hypothyroid patients, before and after treatment. *J. Clin. Endocrin.* 27:1593–99.

Kales, A.; Hoedemacher, F. S.; Jacobson, A.; and Lichtenstein, E. L. 1964. Dream deprivation: an experimental reappraisal. *Nature* 204:1337–38.

Kales, A.; Kales, J. D.; Scharf, M. B.; and Tan, T. L. 1970. Hypnotics and altered sleep-dream patterns. II. All-night EEG studies of chloral hydrate, flurazepam, and metaqualone. *Arch. Gen. Psychiat.* 23:219–25.

Kales, A.; Tan, T. L.; Kollar, E. J.; Naitoh, P.; Preston, T. A.; and Malmstrom, E. J. 1970. Sleep patterns following 205 hours of sleep deprivation. *Psychosom. Med.* 32:189–200.

Kant, I. 1966. *Critique of Pure Reason.* New York: Anch. Doubleday.

Karacan, I.; Goodenough, D.; Shapiro, A.; and Starker, S. 1966. Erection cycle during sleep in relation to dream anxiety. *Arch. Gen. Psychiat.* 15:183–89.

Kawamura, H., and Sawyer, C. 1964. D. C. Potential changes in the rabbit during slow-wave and paradoxical sleep. *Amer. J. Physiol.* 207:1379–86.

Kety, S. S. 1970. The biogenic amines in the central nervous system: their possible roles in arousal, emotion, and learning. In *The Neurosciences Second Study Program*, ed. F. O. Schmitt, G. C. Quarton, T. Melnechuk, and G. Adelman, pp. 324–36. New York: Rockefeller.

King, C. D. 1972. The pharmacology of rapid eye movement sleep. *Advan. Pharmacol. Chemother.* 9:1–91.

Klein, M.; Michel, F.; and Jouvet, M. 1964. Etude polygraphique de sommeil chez les oisseaux. *C.R. Soc. Biol.* 158:99–103.

Kleitman, N. 1927. Studies on the physiology of sleep. V. Some experiments on puppies. *Amer. J. Physiol.* 84:386–95.

Kleitman, N. 1963. *Sleep and Wakefulness*, 2nd ed. Chicago: U. of Chicago Pr.

Kleitman, N., and Kleitman, H. 1953. The sleep-wakefulness pattern in the Arctic. *Scientific Monthly* 76:349–56.

Kline, N. 1958. Clinical experience with iproniazid (Marsilid). *J. Clin. Exp. Psychopath.* 19(suppl.):72–79.

Koella, W. P. 1967. *Sleep: Its Nature and Physiological Organization.* Springfield, Ill.: Charles C. Thomas.

Koella, W. P.; Feldstein, A.; and Czicman, J. 1968. The effect of parachlorophenylalanine on the sleep of cats. *Electroencephalog. Clin. Neurophysiol.* 25:481–90.

Kollar, E. J.; Pasnau, R. O.; Rubin, R. T.; Naitoh, P.; Slater, G. G.; and Kales, A. 1969. Psychologic, psychophysiologic, and biochemical correlates of prolonged sleep deprivation. *Amer. J. Psychiat.* 126:488–97.

Kuhn, D. J.; Meltzer, H. Y.; Wyatt, R. J.; and Snyder, F. 1970. Serum enzyme changes during sleep deprivation. *Nature* 228:768–69.

Kuhn, E.; Brodan, V.; Brodanova, M.; and Friedman, B. 1967. Influence of sleep deprivation on iron metabolism. *Nature* 213:1041–42.

Kulkarni, A. S. 1968. Facilitation of instrumental avoidance learning by amphetamine: an analysis. *Psychopharmacologia* 13:418–25.

Latz, A.; Bain, G.; Goldman, M.; and Kornetsky, C. 1967. Maze learning after administration of antidepressant drugs. *J. Pharmacol. Exp. Ther.* 156:76–84.

Leconte, P., and Bloch, V. 1970. Deficit de la retention d'un conditionnement après privation de sommeil paradoxal chez la rat. *C.R. Acad. Sci.* 271:226–29.

Leconte, P.; Hennevin, E.; and Bloch, V. 1972. Increase in paradoxical sleep following learning in the rat: correlation with level of conditioning. *Brain Res.* 42:552–53.

Lewin, B. D. 1950. *The Psychoanalysis of Elation.* New York: Norton.

Lewin, I., and Gombosh, D. 1972. Increase in REM time as a function of the need for divergent thinking. Report to the First European Congress of Sleep Research, October 3–6, Basel, Switzerland.

Lewis, H. E., and Masterton, J. P. 1957. Sleep and wakefulness in the Arctic. *The Lancet* 1:1262–66.

Lowy, F. H.; Cleghorn, J. M.; and Mc Clure, D. J. 1971. Sleep patterns in depression. *J. Nerv. Ment. Dis.* 153:10–26.

Lucero, M. A. 1970. Lengthening of REM sleep duration consecutive to learning in the rat. *Brain Res.* 20:319–22.

McCarley, R. W., and Hobson, J. A. 1971. Single neuron activity in cat giganto-cellular tegmental field: selectivity of discharge in desynchronized sleep. *Science* 174:1250–55.

MacCurdy, J. T. 1920. The psychology and treatment of insomnia in fatigue and allied states. *J. Abnorm. Psychol.* 15:45–54.

McGinty, D. J. 1969. Effects of prolonged isolation and subsequent enrichment of sleep patterns in kittens. *Electroencephalog. Clin. Neurophysiol.* 26: 332–37.

MacKinnon, I.; MacKinnon, P.; and Thomason, A. 1959. Lethal hazards of the luteal phase of the menstrual cycle. *Brit. Med. J.* 1:1015–17.

Maeder, A. E. 1916. The dream problem. *J. Nerv. Ment. Dis.* Monograph 22.

Mahl, G.; Rothenberg, A.; Delgado, J.; and Hamlin, H. 1961. Psychological responses in the human to intracerebral electrical stimulation. *Psychosom. Med.* 26:337–68.

Mangold, R.; Sokoloff, L.; Conner, E.; Kleinerman, J.; Therman, P. -O. G.; and Kety, S. S. 1955. The effects of sleep and lack of sleep on cerebral circulation and metabolism of normal young men. *J. Clin. Invest.* 34:1092–100.

Matsumoto, M.; Nishisho, T.; Sudo, T.; Sadahiro, T.; and Miyoshi, M. 1968. Influence of fatigue on sleep. *Nature* 218:177–78.

Meier, B. W., and Berger, R. J. 1965. Development of sleep and wakefulness patterns in the infant rhesus monkey. *Exp. Neurol.* 12:257–77.

Mendels, J., and Hawkins, D. R. 1967. Sleep and depression: a controlled EEG study. *Arch. Gen. Psychiat.* 16:344–54.

Meyerhoff, J. L., and Snyder, S. H. 1972. Amphetamine isomers in "maladie des tics." *Scientific Proceedings* (in summary form) of the 125th Annual Meeting of the American Psychiatric Association, May, Dallas, Texas.

Monnier, M., and Hosli, L. 1964. Dialysis of sleep and waking factors in blood of the rabbit. *Science* 146:796–98.

Monnier, M., and Hosli, L. 1965. Humoral transmission of sleep and wakefulness. II. Hemodialysis of sleep inducing humor during stimulation of the thalamic somnogenic area. *Arch. Ges. Physiol.* 282:60–75.

Morgan, B. B., Jr.; Brown, B. R.; and Alluisi, E. A. 1970. Effects of 48 hours of continuous work and sleep loss on sustained performance. Department of the Army *Interim Technical Report* no. IRT-70-16, September.

Morris, J. M. 1967. *Fatigue Fractures.* Springfield, Ill.: Charles C. Thomas.

Morton, J.; Additon, H.; Addison, R.; Hunt, L.; and Sullivan, J. 1953. Clinical study of premenstrual tension. *Amer. J. Obstet. Gynec.* 65:1182–91.

Moruzzi, G. 1962–63. Active processes in the brain stem during sleep. *Harvey Lect.* 58:233–97.

Moruzzi, G. 1966. The functional significance of sleep with particular regard to the brain mechanisms underlying consciousness. In *Brain Mechanisms and Conscious Experience*, ed. J. C. Eccles, pp. 345–88. New York: Springer-Verlag.

Moruzzi, G., and Magoun, H. 1949. Brain stem reticular formation and activation of the EEG. *Electroencephalog. Clin. Neurophysiol.* 1:455–73.

Mouret, J.; Bobiller, P.; and Jouvet, M. 1967. Effets de la parachlorophenylalanine sur le sommeil du rat. *C.R. Soc. Biol.* 161:1600–03.

Naitoh, P. 1969. Sleep loss and its effects on performance. U.S. Navy Medical Neuropsychiatric Research Unit, report no. 68–3. Rept./21–51.

Naitoh, P.; Johnson, L. C.; and Lubin, A. 1971. Modification of surface negative slow potential (CNV) in the human brain after total sleep loss. *Electroencephalog. Clin. Neurophysiol.* 30:17–22.

Naitoh, P.; Kales, A.; Kollar, E. J.; Smith, J. C.; and Jacobson, A. 1969. Electroencephalographic activity after prolonged sleep loss. *Electroencephalog. Clin. Neurophysiol.* 27:2–11.

Naitoh, P.; Pasnau, R. O.; and Kollar, E. J. 1971. Psychophysiological changes after prolonged deprivation of sleep. *Biol. Psychiat.* 3:309–20.

Naitoh, P., and Townsend, R. E. 1970. The role of sleep deprivation research in human factors. *Human Factors* 12:575–85.

Newman, E. A., and Evans, C. R. 1965. Human dream processes as analogous to computer programme clearance. *Nature* 206:534.

Noda, H., and Adey, W. R. 1970. Firing of neuron pairs in cat association cortex during sleep and wakefulness. *J. Neurophysiol.* 33:672–84.

Oliverio, A. 1965. Neurohumoral systems and learning. In *Psychopharmacology: A Review of Progress 1957–1967*, ed. L. Goodman and A. Gilman. 3rd ed. New York: Macmillan.

Oswald, I. 1970. Sleep, the great restorer. *New Scientist* 46:170–72.

Oswald, I. 1972. Report to the First European Congress of Sleep Research, October 3–6, Basel, Switzerland.

Oswald, I.; Berger, R. J.; Jaramillo, R. A.; Keddie, K. M. G.; Olley, P. C.; and Plunkett, G. B. 1963. Melancholia and barbiturates: a controlled EEG, body and eye movement study of sleep. *Brit. J. Psychiat.* 109:66–78.

Pappenheimer, J. R.; Miller, T. B.; and Goodrich, C. A. 1967. Sleep-promoting effects of cerebrospinal fluid from sleep-deprived goats. *Proc. Nat. Acad. Sci. USA* 58:513–17.

Parmalee, A.; Schulz, H.; and Disbrow, M. 1961. Sleep patterns of the newborn. *J. Pediat.* 58:241–50.

Passouant, P.; Cadilhac, J.; Delange, M.; Callamand, M.; and Kasabgui, E. 1964. Age et sommeil: variations electrocliniques du sommeil, de la naissance a l'extreme vieillesse. *Rev. Neurol.* 110:303–04.

Passouant, P.; Passouant-Fontaine, T.; and Cadilhac, J. 1966. L'influence de hyperthyroidie sur le sommeil etude clinique et experimentale. *Rev. Neurol.* 115:353–66.

Pavlov, I. P. 1952. The sleep problem. *Feldsher Akush.* 8:3–7; 9:3–7; 10:3–5.

Pearlman, C. 1970. The adaptive function of dreaming. In *Sleep and Dreaming*, ed. E. Hartmann, International Psychiatry Clinics Series, vol. 7, pp. 329–34. Boston: Little, Brown.

Pearlman, C., and Greenberg, R. 1968. Effect of REM deprivation on retention of avoidance learning in rats. Report to the 8th Annual Meeting of the Association for the Psychophysiological Study of Sleep, March, Denver, Colorado.

Pegram, V.; Hammond, D.; and Bridgers, W. 1972. The effect of protein synthesis inhibition on sleep in the mouse. Report to the 11th Annual Meeting of the Association for the Phychophysiological Study of Sleep, May, Lake Minnewaska, New York. Abstract in *Sleep Research 1971–1972*, ed. M. Chase, W. Stern, and P. Walter. Los Angeles: Brain Information Service, UCLA.

Penfield, W., and Jasper, H. 1954. *Epilepsy and Functional Anatomy of the Human Brain.* Boston: Little, Brown.

Pflug, B., and Toelle, R. 1971. Therapie endogener Depressionen durch Schlafentzug: Praktische und theoretische Konsequenzen. *Nervenarzt* 42:117–24.

Pieron, H. 1913. *Le Probleme Physiologique du Sommeil.* Paris: Masson.

Platman, D., and Fieve, R. Unpublished studies. Personal communication to the author.

Pompeiano, O. 1967. The neurophysiological mechanisms of the postural and motor events during desynchronized sleep. In *Sleep and Altered States of Consciousness*, ed. S. S. Kety, E. V. Evarts, and H. L. Williams, pp. 351–423. Baltimore: Williams and Wilkins.

Pompeiano, O. 1970. Mechanisms of sensorimotor integration during sleep. In *Progress in Physiological Psychology*, ed. E. Stellar and J. M. Sprague, vol. 3, pp. 1–79. New York and London: Acad. Pr.

Prechtl, H. F. R. 1970. Brain and behavioral mechanisms in the human newborn infant. In *Brain and Early Behavior*, ed. R. Robinson, pp. 115–38. New York: Acad. Pr.

Pujol, J. F.; Mouret, J.; Jouvet, M.; and Glowinski, J. 1968. Increased turnover of cerebral norepinephrine during rebound of paradoxical sleep in the rat. *Science* 159:112–14.

Rakestraw, N. W., and Whittier, F. O. 1923. The effect of loss of sleep on the composition of the blood and urine. *Proc. Soc. Exp. Biol. Med.* 21:5–6.

Rapaport, D. 1950. The autonomy of the ego. *Bull. Menninger Clinic* 15:113–23.

Rapaport, D. 1951. Toward a theory of thinking. In *Organization and Pathology of Thought*, pp. 689–730. New York: Columbia U. Pr.

Rechtschaffen, A., and Kales, A., eds. 1968. *The Manual of Standardized Terminology, Techniques and Scoring System for Sleep Stages of Human Subjects.* National Institutes of Health Publication no. 204.

Rechtschaffen, A., and Verdone, P. 1964. Amount of dreaming: effect of incentive, adaptation to laboratory, and individual differences. *Percept. Motor Skills* 19:947–58.

Regestein, Q. R., and Hartmann, E. 1972. Unpublished studies.

Reich, P.; Driver, J. K.; and Karnovsky, M. L. 1967. Sleep: effects on incorporation of inorganic phosphate into brain fractions. *Science* 157:336–38.

Reich, P.; Geyer, S. J.; and Karnovsky, M. L. 1972. Metabolism of brain during sleep and wakefulness. *J. Neurochem.* 19:487–98.

Robinson, M. F., and Freeman, W. 1954. *Psychosurgery and the Self.* New York: Grune.

Roffwarg, H.; Muzio, J.; and Dement, W. 1966. Ontogenetic development of human sleep-dream cycle. *Science* 152:604–18.

Rojas-Ramirez, J. A., and Tauber, E. S. 1970. Paradoxical sleep in two species of avian predator (Falconiformes). *Science* 167:1754–55.

Sampson, H. 1966. Psychological effects of deprivation of dreaming sleep. *J. Nerv. Ment. Dis.* 143:305–17.

Sassin, J. F.; Parker, D. C.; Mace, J. W.; Gotlin, R. W.; Johnson, L. C.; and Rossman, L. G. 1969. Human growth hormone release: relation to slow-wave sleep and sleep-waking cycles. *Science* 165:513–15.

Schildkraut, J. J., and Hartmann, E. 1972. Turnover and metabolism of norepinephrine in rat brain after 72 hours on a D-deprivation island. *Psychopharmacologia* 27:17–27.

Schildkraut, J. J., and Kety, S. S. 1967. The biogenic amines and emotion. *Science* 156:21–30.

Schildkraut, J. J.; Schanberg, S.; Breese, G.; and Kopin, I. 1967. Norepinephrine metabolism and drugs used in the affective disorders: A possible mechanism of action. *Amer. J. Psychiat.* 124:600–08.

Seashore, R., and Ivy, A. 1953. Effects of amphetamine drugs in relieving fatigue. *Psychol. Monogr.*, whole no. 365, 67:1–16.

Segal, D. S., and Mandell, A. J. 1970. Behavioral activation of rats during intraventricular infusion of norepinephrine. *Proc. Nat. Acad. Sci.* 66:289–93.

Segal, M.; Disterhoft, J. F.; and Olds, J. 1972. Hippocampal unit activity during classical aversive and appetitive conditioning. *Science* 175:792–94.

Seham, M., and Seham, G. 1926. *The Tired Child.* Philadelphia: Lippincott.

Seiden, L., and Peterson, D. 1968. Reversal of the reserpine-induced suppression of the conditioned avoidance response by l-DOPA: correlation of behavioral and biochemical differences in two strains of mice. *J. Pharmacol. Exp. Ther.* 159:422–28.

Shakespeare, W. 1623. *The Tragedy of Macbeth.* In *The Plays of William Shakespeare.* First Folio Edition. London.

Shapot, V. S. 1957. Brain metabolism in relation to the functional state of central nervous system. In *Metabolsim of the Nervous System,* ed. D. Richter, pp. 257–62. New York: Pergamon.

Sherrington, C. S. 1906. The integrative action of the nervous system. In *Silliman Lectures.* New Haven: Yale U. Pr.

Small, A.; Hibi, S.; and Feinberg, I. 1971. Effects of dextroamphetamine sulfate on EEG sleep patterns of hyperactive children. *Arch. Gen. Psychiat.* 25:369–80.

Snyder, F. 1964. The REM state in a living fossil. Report to the Association for the Psychophysiological Study of Sleep, March, Palo Alto, California.

Snyder, F. 1966. Toward an evolutionary theory of dreaming. *Amer. J. Psychiat.* 123:121–36.

Snyder, F. 1967. In quest of dreaming. In *Experimental Studies of Dreaming,* ed. H. A. Witkin and H. B. Lewis, pp. 3–75. New York: Random.

Snyder, F. 1969. Dynamic aspects of sleep disturbances in relation to mental illness. *Biol. Psychiat.* 1:119–30.

Snyder, F.; Hobson, J.; Morrison, D.; and Goldfrank, F. 1964. Changes in respiration, heart rate and systolic blood pressure in relation to electroencephalographic patterns of human sleep. *J. Appl. Physiol.* 19:417–22.

Spitz, R. A.; Emde, R. N.; and Metcalf, D. R. 1970. Further prototypes of ego formation: a working paper from a research project on early development. In *The Psychoanalytic Study of the Child,* ed. R. S. Eissler et al., pp. 417–41. New York: Intl. Univs. Pr.

Stein, L. 1965. Chemistry of reward and punishment. In *Psychopharmacology: A Review of Progress 1957–1967,* ed. D. Efron. New York: Macmillan.

Stein, L. 1967. Noradrenergic substrates of positive reinforcement: site of motivational action of amphetamine and chlorpromazine. In *Proceedings Fifth Congress Collegium Internationale Neuro-Psycho-Pharmacologicum,* ed. H. Brill, J. Cole, P. Deniker, H. Hippius, and P. Bradley, Washington, D.C., p. 765. International Congress Series no. 129. Amsterdam: Excerpta Medica Foundation.

Stern, M.; Fram, D. H.; Wyatt, R.; Grinspoon, L.; and Tursky, B.

1969. All-night sleep studies of acute schizophrenics. *Arch. Gen. Pschiat.* 20:470–77.

Stern, W. C. 1969*a*. Pharmacological modification of the effects of REM sleep deprivation upon active and passive avoidance in the rat. *Psychophysiology* 6:224.

Stern, W. C. 1969*b*. Behavioral and biochemical aspects of rapid eye movement deprivation in the rat. Ph.D. Diss., Univ. Indiana.

Stern, W. C. 1970. The relationship between REM sleep and learning: animal studies. In *Sleep and Dreaming*, ed. E. Hartmann, International Psychiatry Clinics Series, vol. 7, pp. 249–57. Boston: Little, Brown.

Stern, W. C., and Hartmann, E. 1972. Reduced amphetamine lethality following chronic stress. *Psychopharmacologia* 23:167–70.

Stern, W. C.; Hartmann, E.; Draskoczy, P. R.; and Schildkraut, J. J. 1972. Behavioral effects of centrally administered 6-hydroxydopamine. *Psychol. Rep.* 30:815–20.

Stern, W. C., and Morgane, P. J. 1971. Effects of electrical stimulation of the brain upon subsequent sleep in the cat. Report to the First European Congress of the Association for the Psychophysiological Study of Sleep, June, Bruges, Belgium.

Stern, W. C.; Morgane, P. J.; Panksepp, J.; Zolovick, A. J.; and Jalowiec, J. E. 1972. Elevation of REM sleep following inhibition of protein synthesis. *Brain. Res.* 47:254–58.

Strom-Olsen, R., and Weil-Malherbe, H. 1958. Humoral changes in manic-depressive psychosis with particular reference to the excretion of catecholamines in urine. *J. Ment. Sci.* 104:696–704.

Tagney, J. 1972. Rearing in an enriched or isolated environment: sleep patterns in the rat. Report to the 11th Annual Meeting of the Association for the Psychophysiological Study of Sleep, May, Lake Minnewaska, New York. Abstract in *Sleep Research 1971–1972*, ed. M. Chase, W. Stern, and P. Walter, p. 121. Los Angeles: Brain Information Service, UCLA.

Takahashi, Y.; Kipnis, D. M.; and Daughaday, W. H. 1968. Growth hormone secretion during sleep. *J. Clin. Invest.* 47:2079–90.

Tauber, E. S.; Rojas-Ramirez, J.; and Hernandez-Peon, R. 1968. Electrophysiological and behavioral correlates of wakefulness and sleep in the lizard, *Ctenosaura pectinata. Electroencephalog. Clin. Neurophysiol.* 27:605–06.

Tecce, J. J. 1972. Contingent negative variation (CNV) and psychological processes in man. *Psychol. Bull.* 77:73–108.

Torda, C. 1969. Dreams of subjects with loss of memory for recent events. *Psychophysiology* 6:352–65.

Tyler, D. B. 1955. Psychological changes during experimental sleep deprivation. *Dis. Nerv. Syst.* 14:293–99.

Tyler, D. B.; Goodman, J.; and Rothman, T. 1947. The effect of experimental insomnia on the rate of potential changes in the brain. *Amer. J. Physiol.* 149:185–93.

Uretsky, N. J., and Iversen, L. L. 1969. Effects of 6-hydroxydopamine on noradrenaline-containing neurones in the rat brain. *Nature* 221:557–59.

Valatx, J. L. 1972. Report to the First European Congress of Sleep Research, October 3–6, Basel, Switzerland.

Vander Wolf, C. H. 1969. Hippocampal electrical activity and voluntary movement in the rat. *Electroencephalog. Clin. Neurophysiol.* 26:407–18.

Verdone, P. 1965. Temporal reference of manifest dream content. *Percept. Motor Skills* 20:1253–68.

Verdone, P. 1968. Sleep satiation: extended sleep in normal subjects. *Electroencephalog. Clin. Neurophysiol.* 24:417–23.

Villablanca, J. 1972. Permanent reduction in sleep after removal of cerebral cortex and striatum in cats. *Brain Res.* 36:463–68.

Vital-Durand, F., and Michel, F. 1971. Effets de la désafferentiation péripherique sur le cycle veille-sommeil chez le chat. *Arch. Ital. Biol.* 109:166–86.

Vogel, G. W. 1968. REM deprivation. III. Dreaming and psychosis. *Arch. Gen. Psychiat.* 18:312–29.

Vogel, G. W., and Traub, A. C. 1968. REM deprivation. I. The effect on schizophrenic patients. *Arch. Gen. Psychiat.* 18:287–300.

Vogel, G. W.; Traub, A. C.; Ben-Horin, P.; and Meyers, G. M. 1968. REM deprivation. II. The effects on depressed patients. *Arch. Gen. Psychiat.* 18:301–11.

Walter, W. G. 1964. The contingent negative variation: an electrocortical sign of significant association in the human brain. *Science* 146:434.

Watson, R. 1972. Mental correlates of periobarbital: phasic integrated potentials during REM sleep. Ph.D. thesis, Univ. Chicago.

Watson, R.; Hartmann, E.; and Schildkraut, J. J. 1972. Amphetamine withdrawal: affective state, sleep patterns, and MHPG excretion. *Amer. J. Psychiat.* 129:263–69.

Webb, W. B. 1961. An overview of sleep as an experimental variable 1940–1959. *Science* 134:1421–23.

Webb, W. B. 1962. Some effects of prolonged sleep deprivation on the hooded rat. *J. Comp. Physiol. Psychol.* 55:791–93.

Webb, W. B. 1969. Twenty-four-hour sleep cycling. In *Sleep: Physiology and Pathology, A Symposium*, ed. A. Kales, pp. 53–65. Philadelphia: Lippincott.

Webb, W. B. 1971. Paper presented at a symposium of the First International Congress of the Association for the Psychophysiological Study of Sleep, June, Bruges, Belgium.

Webb, W. B., and Agnew, H. W., Jr. 1970. Sleep stage characteristics of long and short sleepers. *Science* 168:146–47.

Webb, W. B., and Freidman, J. 1971. Attempts to modify the sleep patterns of the rat. *Physiol. Behav.* 6:459–60.

Weiss, B., and Laties, V. 1962. Enhancement of human performance by caffeine and the amphetamines. *Pharmacol. Rev.* 14:1–36.

Weiss, T. 1966. Discussion of "The D-state" by E. Hartmann. *Int. J. Psychiat.* 2:32–36.

Weiss, T., and Roldan, E. 1964. Comparative study of sleep cycles in rodents. *Experientia* 20:280–81.

Wender, P. H. 1971. *Minimal Brain Dysfunction in Children.* New York: Wiley.

West, L. J.; Janszen, H. H.; Lester, B. K.; and Cornelison, F. S. 1962. The psychosis of sleep deprivation. *Ann. N.Y. Acad. Sci.* 98:66–79.

Wilkinson, R. T. 1964. Artifical "signals" as an aid to an inspection task. *Ergonomics* 7:63–72.

Wilkinson, R. T. 1965. Sleep deprivation. In *The Physiology of Human Survival*, ed. O. G. Edholm and A. L. Bacharach, pp. 399–429. New York: Acad. Pr.

Wilkinson, R. T. 1970. Methods for research on sleep deprivation and sleep function. In *Sleep and Dreaming*, ed. E. Hartmann, International Psychiatry Clinics Series, vol. 7, pp. 369–81. Boston: Little, Brown.

Wilkinson, R. T.; Edwards, R. S.; and Haines, E. 1966. Performance following a night of reduced sleep. *Psychonom. Sci.* 5:471–72.

Williams, D. H., and Cartwright, R. D. 1969. Blood pressure changes during EEG-monitored sleep. *Arch. Gen. Psychiat.* 20:307–14.

Williams, H. L.; Hammack, J. T.; Daly, R. L.; Dement, W. C.; and Lubin, A. 1964. Responses to auditory stimulation, sleep loss, and

EEG stages of sleep. *Electroencephalog. Clin. Neurophysiol.* 16:269–79.

Williams, H. L.; Lubin, A.; and Goodnow, J. J. 1959. Impaired performance with acute sleep loss. *Psychol. Mongr.*: General and Applied 73:1–26.

Witkin, H. A., and Lewis, H. B. 1967. Presleep experiences and dreams. In *Experimental Studies of Dreaming*, ed. H. A. Witkin and H. B. Lewis, pp. 148–225. New York: Random.

Wohlisch, E. 1956. Schlaf und Erholung als Proleme der Energetik und Gefassversorgung des Gehirns. *Klin. Wschr.* 34:720–29.

Wolff, P. H. 1966. The causes, controls, and organization of behavior in the neonate. *Psychol. Issues* 5:1–105.

Wolff, W. 1952. *The Dream-Mirror of Conscience.* New York: Grune.

Wyatt, R. J.; Chase, T. N.; Scott, J.; and Snyder, F. 1970. Effect of l-DOPA on the sleep of man. *Nature* 228:999–1000.

Wyatt, R. J.; Kupfer, D. J.; Scott, J.; Robinson, D. S.; and Snyder, F. 1969. Longitudinal studies of the effect of monoamine oxidase inhibitors on sleep in man. *Psychopharmacologia* 15:236–44.

Zimmerman, J.; Stoyva, J.; and Metcalf, D. 1969. Distorted visual experience and rapid eye movement sleep. Report to the 9th Annual Meeting of the Association for the Psychophysiological Study of Sleep, March, Boston, Mass.

Zung, W. W. K. 1969. Antidepressant drugs and sleep. *Exp. Med. Surg.* 27:124–37.

Zung, W. W. K.; Wilson, W. P.; and Dodson, W. E. 1964. Effect of depressive disorders on sleep EEG responses. *Arch. Gen. Psychiat.* 10:439–45.

INDEX

Active sleep. *See* D-sleep
Adaptation: and selection, 15, 28; psychological, 17; to environment, 157
Adaptive ego mechanisms, 156
Adaptive point of view, 129
Age: and sleep, 15, 18, 82–87; and neurophysiological processes, 83; curves for sleep variables, 83–86
Alpha-methylparatyrosine. *See* AMPT
Alpha waves, 23, 41
Amitriptyline, 106n3, 112. *See also* Antidepressant medication
Amphetamines, 112; and sleep deprivation, 42, 113; withdrawal from, 92–93, 109; and alertness, 113; and catecholamines, 113, 157; and performance, 114; and attention, 115; and secondary process, 115; and "need to achieve," 115; paradoxical effect, 115; counteracting sleep deprivation, 116; lethality in animals, 116–17; and hyperkinetic child, 117; and D-sleep, 117; psychological effect, 154–55
Amphibians: sleep in, 27
AMPT, 107, 112; and D-sleep, 107–08, 119; and waking, 119; and learning deficit, 120
Anabolism: and sleep, 88, 151
Anger: and sleep deprivation, 44, 45; and sleep requirement, 78
Antidepressant medication, 105–06, 109, 121, 149
Antigravity muscles, 26
Anxiety: and sleep requirement, 69, 77, 89–90, 94
Apes: sleep in, 28
Aphasia: and sleep, 88–89
Arousal: function of D-sleep, 12–13; during S- and D-sleep, 13; systems, 16; threshold, 26

Attention, 156–59; after sleep deprivation, 43; and sleep, 51; narrowed, 115; and tiredness, 127; processes in dreams, 137; repaired during dreaming, 140
Auld scale, 64
Autonomic functions, 10
Autonomic nervous system: and sleep deprivation, 42
Awakenings, nature of, 26–27

Basal metabolic rate, 28–30, 84
Benzodiazepines: and slow-wave sleep, 106
Binocular vision, 15, 17
Biogenic amines, 35, 107; and convulsion threshold, 119. *See also* Catecholamines
Birds: sleep in, 27, 37
Blood chemistry: effect of sleep deprivation on, 41
Blood metabolites, 7
Blood pressure: during sleep, 24
Brain: chemistry, 35; oxygen consumption, 84; stimulation, 102–03; pathways, interconnections between, 133; systems and psychology, 159, 161–63; as organ of adaptation, 162; and ego, 162, 164
Brain stem, 32
Buffering: in tiredness, 129

California Personality Inventory (CPI), 58, 63, 64
Carnivores: sleep in, 28
Catabolism: and slow-wave sleep, 94
Catecholamines, 35; functions, 11–16, 154–59; and D-deprivation, 50–51; and D-sleep, 106–16 passim, 148, 150, 154; and mental illness, 113–14, 158; and motor activity, 114, 154; role in learning, 114, 156; in reward system, 115, 156; and